EXQUISITE MOMENTS *of* SORROW *and* GRACE

KENNETH R. WEINBERG, MD

Book Design and Interior by Kat Hargrave

Printed in the United States of America

First Printing, 2025

ISBN (hardcover) 979-8-9925733-0-5

ISBN (paperback) 979-8-9925733-1-2

ISBN (eBook) 979-8-9925733-2-9

The following stories were previously published in a different version:

"The Man Who Hugged Me,"
The Journal of Emergency Medicine, Vol. 24. No. 3, pp. 347-348, 2003 (with accompanying editorial article/review)

"Study of the Physician as Patient"
(published as "The Physician as Patient"),
Journal of Holistic Healthcare, Vol 3, Issue 4 pp. 7-10, 2006

"Always a Doctor, Even in the Dying of the Light."
The New York Times / Science Times, "Cases" section. October 14, 2008

"The Little Nowhere of the Mind,"
Intima: A Journal of Narrative Medicine, September 2012

"Wind Tunnel,"
Intima: A Journal of Narrative Medicine, Spring 2017

"Schmeckle Down,"
Intima: A Journal of Narrative Medicine, Fall 2020

"Fucking Headache,"
Intima: A Journal of Narrative Medicine, Fall 2023

DEDICATION

For Georgia, and Susan

"There are no diseases, only patients."

—Sir William Osler,
co-founding professor
of Johns Hopkins Hospital

EARLY PRAISE FOR *EXQUISITE MOMENTS OF SORROW AND GRACE*

"Reading these stories brought me right back to Bellevue's ER, the feelings and the sounds, the sights and smells. Weinberg has a gift for weaving a tapestry of patient tales while pulling on our heartstrings."

—*Julie Holland MD, and author,* Weekends at Bellevue, Nine Years on the Night Shift at the Psych ER *(Random House)*

"In *Exquisite Moments of Sorrow and Grace*, Dr. Kenneth Weinberg invites readers on a powerful journey that renders them to consider what truly sets a great doctor apart. Drawing on 40 years in the ER, he reveals how effective medicine demands a deft balance of compassion, clinical judgment, and seamless collaboration. With clarity and heart, Dr. Weinberg illustrates how intuition, science, and situational awareness guide seasoned professionals through high-stakes decisions. Weinberg's stories of heartbreak, joy, shock, and relief expose the mental and emotional agility required of ER staff. More than a memoir, this book offers insight into the human side of healing—and the profound capacities of compassionate care."

—*Maggie C. Vaughan, LMFT, PhD, founder and director, Happy Apple* NYC

"*Exquisite Moments of Sorrow and Grace* is a beautifully written and deeply moving work that captures the complexities of the human experience. The author reveals an emotional depth which stays with you long after reading, offering both moments of heartbreak and unexpected solace. The themes of love, loss, resilience, and redemption are woven together masterfully. This book will not only challenge you but also, leave you with a greater appreciation for the fragile beauty of life."

—*Angelique Khalifa, Ph.D., toxicologist*

"As a grateful recipient of both a heart and kidney transplant, I truly appreciated Dr. Weinberg's insightful commentary on some of the most critical medical moments."

—*Jerry Libbin, author of* Chambers of the Heart: Strategies for Thriving in Life and Business

"Dr. Weinberg's *Exquisite Moments of Sorrow and Grace* offers an honest, even charming, look into the realities of emergency room medicine and mental health. He illuminates the vital role of human connection and grace especially during stressful experiences. These stories serve as a powerful reminder that medicine is not merely a science, but an art, where empathy and compassion are essential tools for healing. Weinberg's work underscores the importance of the doctor-patient relationship, highlighting how genuine human interaction can provide comfort and support during times of crisis."

—*Amy Henry, author of* Big Desire *and creator of The Desire Method*

"It is rare to come across a book that blends the rigor of medicine with the tenderness of human experience as masterfully as *Exquisite Moments of Sorrow and* Grace, by Dr. Kenneth R. Weinberg. His clinical recollections, drawn from the frontlines of emergency medicine, go far beyond technical narratives—they are profound reflections on life, vulnerability, and the quiet courage found in moments of crisis. As someone who witnesses the daily challenges of public health from a global perspective, I regard this work as an essential international reference. Dr. Weinberg's writing transcends borders. It speaks to all of us—physicians, communicators, caregivers, and citizens—who believe in the power of empathy, attentive care, and human dignity. Dr. Weinberg is a storyteller of the soul."

—*Claudia Cataldi, president, Brazilian Association of Electronic and Digital Media Press, director of communication and marketing, Rede Governança Brasil and Brazilian War College Alumni*

"This is a fascinating memoir of the chaotic rhythms of an ER physician's life with the fullness of a personal story woven within the countless hours of a focused healer. Human nature expressions from his personal story within family memories and of the extremely tense moments of an ordinary day in an emergency department make for a riveting exposé of life for many physicians, physician assistants and nurses who risk their own health physically and mentally while immersed in this state of adrenaline-pumping emergency. Personal stories like Dr. Weinberg's are necessary and generate a deeper understanding and empathy for the healthcare field within emergency departments everywhere."

—*Diana Devi, yoga teacher and wellness coach, author of* Reach and Receive

CONTENTS

FOREWORD

Ken Weinberg has spent his career in medicine amid large healthcare institutions in Los Angeles and New York. Weinberg practiced emergency medicine in New York City in large hospitals and small hospitals in New Jersey. Weinberg's training in the emergency department (ED) and with Rita Charon, MD, a professor of clinical medicine and director of the program in narrative medicine at the College of Physicians and Surgeons at Columbia, is evident throughout this book. Weinberg has learned to listen to and to observe the most complex of human experiences in the emergency department (ED) and urgent care centers. He demonstrates compassionate, ethical care for patients, often during the worst experiences of their lives.

He teaches us about people, as patients and family members, and describes doctors who are strong and weak and diseases that are simple or very complex. He shows us that the demands of society to make medicine more efficient and particularly faster to save lives, may not be good medicine for some and may be misleading for others.

He has studied the human experience in the emergency department. His writing captures the workers—nurses, emergency medicine technicians, physician's assistants and physicians—in pleasure, doubt, and mostly emphasizes collaboration. Anyone who has worked in an ED will see the characters in the book as real partners in care. This fascinating collection captures the language, meaning, and atmosphere of the emergency department. The relationships of these nurses, emergency medical technicians, physician's assistants and physicians, are seen in every emergency workspace. How these coworkers share anxiety, stress and decision making demonstrates the realities of creating a healthcare team. The conversations show fears, medical errors and joys in saving lives. Several interesting patients and their diseases demonstrate how we learn medicine and the cultural anthropology of the emergency department.

Weinberg's personality and philosophy of medicine are presented in a well-written humanistic fashion. Weinberg is at ease with his patients, the practice of medicine and the task of solving problems and asking questions. He has caught the spirit and narrative of the emergency department and its staff. The lives of emergency department patients and staff are creatively described. This book will be enjoyable for emergency staff and patients—it is the real thing.

—*Lewis R. Goldfrank*, MD, Professor of Emergency Medicine at New York University School of Medicine

CHAPTER 1

Always a Doctor, Even in the Dying of the Light

"Kenny, I want you to see something." As he spoke, my father pulled up a corner of the bandage on his right forearm. I watched a BB-size rent in his skin glisten and begin to bleed.

"Now feel my blood," he told me. "It's cold."

I looked at his face and then back at his arm, unsure how to proceed. The limb was bruised and discolored, damaged by countless needle sticks and transfusions.

We were sitting in the bedroom of his house in Florida. I'd flown down the day before, Sunday, after my mother called to say it appeared that his longstanding, dangerously low blood counts were finally bringing his life to an end.

My brother, Neil, and I had spent the night in his room. We had comforted him when paroxysms of abdominal cramping caused him to cry out as he dozed; we had cleaned him as we silently glanced at each other to confirm that his internal bleeding seemed to have stopped.

Now it was Monday afternoon and with eyes fixed on me, he was talking about how even though he had retired as a physician years before, he still prided himself on keeping up with the latest in medicine. At that moment, it struck me that his body and its skewed hematological functions had become fascinating to him in a detached, scientific way. And I realized there was no way I could refuse his request. I reached my hand out toward the wet circle pooling on his forearm.

"You're right, it is cold," I said, as my finger touched the congealing wound and I tried, in my own scientific way, to figure out how that could be.

"Watch and see what that looks like tomorrow," he announced, the parameters of this latest medical experiment on his body now having been fully defined to his satisfaction.

By Tuesday, my father seemed stable enough for Neil and me to fly home. My brother, Marc, and his son, Ben, came later that day to take up the filial watch. Early Wednesday morning, my father began bleeding again, this time uncontrollably. Marc called the immediate family, and everyone flew down.

When we arrived, Marc told us about the nightmarish vigil he and Ben had just kept. Despite my father's pain, despite a psychic state that had him talking to an unseen man in the room, a man who seemed to be his own father, despite Marc's telling him it was okay to die (a reassurance met with a loud "No!"), despite all this, he spent his last hours refusing to consent to hospice care.

Finally, even he could bear it no longer. He accepted the morphine and the sedative, and his pain abated. My mother lay down next to him, kissed him and told him she loved him. Tears came to his eyes, and he stopped breathing.

As my brothers later told me, both they and my father shared my conviction that his bone marrow failure was caused by his lifelong exposure to radiation; he was a radiologist for fifty years.

Yet he still received marrow-stimulating medications, submitted to transfusions when the drugs failed to work, and kept on moving, defiantly fighting the dying of the light. No longer able to play golf, he plunged into bridge games and kibitzing with his friends in the clubhouse in their community. At his memorial service, we heard how he had pushed to ensure that emergency medical service call buttons were placed throughout the club. Until the week he died, he and I had our Sunday phone conversations about that day's talk shows.

I don't know how he stayed alive so long with blood counts that I, as an emergency physician, associate only with patients at the edge of death. I don't know why his blood felt cold and most of all, I don't know why his dying brought no tears to my eyes. Was it because after his memorial service, determined to celebrate his life, my brothers and I bought champagne and then, at my mother's request, went into his closet, tried on his old clothes and staged a spontaneous fashion show, causing the assembled wives and grandchildren, and my mother, to laugh for an uproarious hour?

Or was it because he died at home, surrounded by those he loved, in such stark contrast to what I experience so often at work: all those patients circling the drain on trips between nursing home and emergency room, and then dying alone with no one to feel their blood turn cold?

CHAPTER 2

Creep and Rainy Day

I never totally understood my parents' relationship. I suppose many kids don't, really.

I do know that the Weinberg and the Vaintrob families lived very close to one another in Newark, starting in the early 1900s and that my father, who was nine years older than my mom, talked about how he'd watched the ambulance come to take my grandmother, Sara Vaintrob, to the hospital to give birth to my very premature mother, and to her twin, who died at birth.

I'd heard that my mother, Renee, had always had a crush on my father and that his mother, Anne, had told him, "When you are ready to settle down, Renee is the girl you should marry."

My father was very good-looking, as well as a bit of a wise guy and womanizer as a younger man, but right after he returned from World War II (he served as a flight surgeon and came home with pilot's wings as a Major), he called my mother and asked, "Are you sitting down?'"

He told her he'd like to take her out on a date. My mother, very smart, artistic, beautiful, and much sought after herself, apparently immediately told him she would be delighted. (I don't know if she was sitting down when she replied.)

They were married two years later.

But I think the fact that she was so much younger, was an only child, and had been quite protected by her parents (they even felt that her commuting to NYU from Newark was too dangerous, so she attended and graduated from Drew University in Madison, New Jersey) were vulnerabilities that she brought to the relationship. My father, on the other hand, was strong-willed, not prone to give in nor admit he could be wrong.

He made us all crazy when we'd go on long road trips by insisting, we could only pull into gas stations that gave out S&H Green Stamps for a fill-up, often forcing us to drive "on fumes" until we found one that did so. He was also in denial about his wise guy side as he was raising us, all the while surreptitiously transmitting this trait to his three (wise guy) sons. This created a dynamic that at times caused issues with my parents.

C. Richard Weinberg, my father, was known by many names. The C stood for Clarence, which my father hated. (His father named him after Clarence Darrow, the famed left-wing, civil liberties lawyer.) Most of his friends called him Clepe, an apparent reference to the Middle English word, yclept, to be called, in Chaucer's Canterbury Tales, a book that he and his buddies enjoyed riffing on in high school. Others called him Dick, or Richard, or, if they thought they knew him but actually didn't, they called him Clete. Years later, my brothers came up with the names "Creep" and "Rainy Day", to characterize my parents.

In any case, Clepe grew up in the bustling city of Newark, New Jersey, in the 1920s and '30s. It was a time before the building of the Holland Tunnel in 1930, linking New Jersey and New York, and Newark still had a very active and distinctive, cultural ambiance. There was a lot of vying for political power among the Jews and Italians and to a lesser extent, the Blacks who all lived in their separate enclaves. There was also a major mob presence as well. Dutch Schulz was gunned down in a Newark tavern in 1935. I think that this all had a significant effect on my father's view of the world.

Many years later, when my parents were living full-time in Florida, I invited Sal Laraia, my primary care doctor, who was then in Boca Raton on vacation, to join us for dinner. A few years prior, I had needed a doctor and, having been very impressed by his medical abilities had asked Sal if he would take me on as a patient. I think that ER docs have the best sense of the abilities, and lack thereof, of the other doctors on staff at the hospitals we work in. The good ones' patients we'd rarely see. The patients of the ones of questionable abilities and ethics would show up regularly under disturbing circumstances. Or those docs would refuse to admit patients when they were on call.

That night in Delray Beach, Sal and his wife came to the house before dinner and I could see that, while my father was being polite and engaging, he clearly thought Sal was a gumba. I was surprised and upset that he was still carrying around that anti-Italian prejudice from his growing up in Newark seventy years prior.

And it seems that Clepe, his relatives, and friends also learned the lingo of the hipsters in that heady time between the wars in the cultural gumbo that Newark was then.

I never considered it unusual that my father and his brother Martin always addressed each other with "Hey, baby!" when meeting, and "Keep the faith," upon departing. But his use of those and other hipster phrases was pointed out to me by a very straight friend in medical school, and it made me aware that that was a significant part of how my father saw himself, even up till the time that he died.

I think it also explained his love of words, Yiddishisms, and made-up expressions. He would often refer to medications he thought were useless as "dreckamine sulfate," dreck being the Yiddish word for shit. People whom he didn't respect were called "Schmegelsky." His colleagues in the medical profession who thought too much of themselves, "schvance melamud," (a learned dick). Any place he considered out in the boonies was called Pennsyltucky. And for some reason (maybe his time at college in Chapel Hill, North Carolina, where he told us of meeting rednecks there who asked if they could feel the back of his head for the horns they'd been told Jews possessed), he nicknamed me and my two best friends, Herkimer, Abner, and Ezekiel. Of course, a few years later, they returned the favor, referring to him thereafter as "Clepshtein." In fact, at my fiftieth birthday party, sitting with Abner and Zeke in my loft in Soho, Clepe was asked by Zeke which of the two of them had been the worst influence on me. (My father had never trusted either of them.) Clepe didn't skip a beat. He turned to Zeke and immediately said, "You were," to Zeke's great astonishment and dismay.

Clepe's father, Mischa, had been a Talmudic scholar in Russia and was apparently descended from the Baal Shem Tov (the 17th-century healer and scholar whose adherents began the Hasidic movement). When Mischa came to New York City (fleeing the pogroms and having become an agnostic), he began working as a motorman on the BMT subway as he put himself through medical school at Fordham University. But, at the same time, apparently, for financial reasons, he felt compelled to place Clepe and his older brother Arthur (named for King Arthur) in a foster home for a few of the years while he was going to school. Clarence and Arthur were very young; it was way out on Long Island. The woman who ran the place was apparently a monster, and my father deeply resented the experience. I always wondered if it was also the reason my father was not particularly studious through high school. He was such an unmotivated student that we were told that Mischa had said Clepe would never make anything of himself, and he'd have to buy him a candy store so he could earn a living.

I never noticed this resentment and anger at his father and yet I will never forget that at Mischa's funeral, I looked up from watching the casket being lowered into the ground and saw my uncle Martin sobbing, overcome with grief, as my father stood by the grave, stone-faced.

While he never really talked about it, and I never thought to ask, I suspect that what finally got my father going was being surrounded by a family whose deep cultural, intellectual, and political interests and influences were very strong. Long before I was born, there was a very active "Cousins Club," with arguments in those days between the pro-Trotsky and pro-Stalin factions. These continued throughout my young adulthood at frequent get-togethers with extended relatives, along with a lot of kibbitzing, respect, and love. In addition, a large contingent of the family (the Seidlers) lived in Detroit. My father eventually went to medical school there at Wayne State and lived with his cousins. Manny Seidler, the head of the family, was a prominent attorney and served as Norman Thomas' campaign manager each time Thomas ran for President on the Socialist Party ticket. Manny ran for the office of Governor of Michigan on that same ticket in 1948. I know my father was deeply influenced by their political beliefs.

Interestingly, one of my much older cousins, Murray Seidler (Manny's son), who was growing up in Detroit when my father was in med school there and who wrote the definitive biography of Thomas, *Respectable Radical*, told my brothers and me years later that my father wasn't circumcised. We were flabbergasted and didn't believe him, but realized that as kids, we'd never noticed. It was only when my father was dying and my brother Neil and I were, late one night, cleaning him up after his most recent episode of internal bleeding, that we looked down and realized Murray was right!

I must wonder if Mischa, who'd escaped Eastern Europe during the 1904 pogrom in Kishinev, Moldova, to come to the United States, felt afraid that if similar events were ever to transpire in his adopted country, he wanted to ensure that his two oldest sons wouldn't be identifiable as Jews by that birthright cleft.

One other thing about Mischa. Growing up we were constantly told that he was an extraordinary diagnostician, extremely astute in his ability to quickly suss out the specific cause of the symptoms any of his patients came in with. I'd spent a fair amount of time in his medical office as a child and remember that in a far corner of the room, he had a large magnifying light with a lens, so he could identify any skin lesions his patients had. During my first year of medical school, I had a dream that I was in his office with both Mischa and my father. I was just learning how to make diagnoses at the time, and in the dream, I asked Mischa how he would approach a patient with a specific set of complaints. He gave me an answer, and I asked,

"But Papa Mischa, what if it wasn't that diagnosis?"

He then told me what he'd do next. We went through this several times until finally, not having an answer for me, he took me to that far corner of the office where the magnifying light was. Only now it was covered by a large cloth. He removed the cloth, revealing the crystal ball that sat beneath it, "In that case," he said, placing his hands on the ball and gazing into it, "I'd look in here for the answer."

After medical school, my father wanted to be a surgeon, but at that time in Newark, there was one Jewish family of surgeons who controlled who would go into that field. And it wasn't the more newly arrived Weinbergs.

Instead, my father, having worked as an X-ray technician in high school, wound up becoming a radiologist (or Roentgenologist as the specialty was initially called, in honor of Willem Roentgen, the discoverer of the X-ray). Because of my father's choice, his older brother Arthur, the smartest of all the three brothers (also interested in becoming a doctor, but whose vision was so bad he couldn't read the medical school texts) became an X-ray tech for the International Ladies Garment Workers Union, and Martin subsequently started a very successful X-ray equipment supply business.

My father ran an increasingly busy radiology practice that eventually took on three partners. As his practice was flourishing in the late '50s, he also became the director of the Radiology Department at Newark City Hospital (also known as Martland Medical Center after Harrison Martland, a Newark pathologist who in 1928, coined the term "Punch Drunk Syndrome." This was the first time the medical world had scrutinized the changes that occurred in the brains of boxers, which predated what we now call traumatic brain injury).

As I was growing up, my father was deeply involved with his medical career. He published countless papers in the radiologic literature, some of which I recently discovered. I was initially upset that we'd never discussed this work when I became a doctor and then realized it was actually his gift to me from beyond the grave. He was the president of the Radiological Society of New Jersey among other honors, and was even, unbeknownst to him, written about in The National Enquirer. My godmother, who was an avid reader of that rag, alerted us, and we got a copy of the paper. On page five was a photo of my father pointing to the abdominal X-ray of a prisoner who'd been a patient at Newark City Hospital. In the shot, my father has his finger pointing to the safety pin that the prisoner had swallowed, and that was now clearly visible, sitting in his stomach.

Clepe maintained an extremely busy schedule between the hospital and his practice when we were growing up, usually working six days a week, fitting in barium enemas and GI series on his patients on Saturday mornings.

He was also a very generous man, outraged by injustice. When Castro took over Cuba in 1959, a legion of physicians, including deposed dictator Batista's personal doctor, fled to New Jersey. Despite being extremely qualified to practice medicine in the US, they were thwarted by the New Jersey State Medical Board from being licensed. My father, then head of the Radiology Department at Newark City Hospital, hired them as X-ray technicians and used his influence to expeditiously get them (re)certified as MDs.

In 1965, the mayor of Newark, Hugh Addonizio, appointed my father Director of Hospitals and Institutions in Newark. Two years later, the Newark riots broke out. (Interestingly, in 1970, Addonizio was sent to prison on a major corruption conviction, an investigation of which began during those '67 riots). Many of my friends' parents were trying to venture to Newark to board up or protect their businesses there during the mayhem. My father, on the other hand wearing a hard hat, was driving back and forth to the hospital from our home in South Orange in an unmarked, black Newark police cruiser with a two-way radio.

Though he never discussed it, he also ran the Emergency Room at Newark City Hospital during the riots, relying on those skills he'd acquired dealing with trauma in World War II. (Amusingly, my best friend, Kenny Weissberg, the one whom he'd nicknamed Abner, wrote his final paper to graduate in 1970 from Wisconsin, on the Newark riots. Amusing to me because he quoted extensively from Dr. C. Richard Weinberg to give the paper immediacy and authenticity, a sense of what it felt like to be an insider at the time. The issue was that Abner knew that no one would ever question the quotes' veracity. He never actually interviewed my father and just made them up to buttress the points he was trying to make. Weissberg reminded me recently that he got an "A" on the paper.)

Clepe also was open-minded in many ways about medicine. When I started to develop myopia, he turned me on to exercises meant to strengthen my eyesight. He talked about *lactobacillus acidophilus* long before it had hit the mainstream as a way of dealing with GI issues and when my brother Neil became an acupuncturist (as opposed to his other two sons who were more mainstream medical practitioners), he was very supportive and often had Neil bring out his acupuncture needles and moxa sticks to treat him for various maladies he had as he got older.

He also had interesting relationships with some of the elderly Eastern European Jews whom he'd run across over the years, including one named Sam Spielberg. Sam would call my father at home and kvetch, all in Yiddish, about being the last remaining white man in Newark, and about the toxicity of the bus fumes where he lived (my brothers and I laughed about that at the time. In retrospect, he clearly was on to something.) My father would sit and listen, a bemused look on his face, and occasionally respond in his own pidgin Yiddish, trying to make Sam feel better.

I realized recently that I had similar relationships with some of my patients, in particular Franklin S. and Harry S., enjoying and being intrigued by their odd observations, mannerisms, and neologisms just like my father did with Sam.

My father became the director of Newark City Hospital after it had lost its residency accreditation and had a terrible reputation. Mayor Addonizio trusted Clepe to regain them again. Within a few years, not only had my father gotten the accreditation back, but he was graduating up to forty residents a year at the program there. It was during this time as well that he was instrumental in wrestling New Jersey College of Medicine out of the hands of the Seton Hall crew running the school in Jersey City and bringing it to Newark. With his usual wisdom and foresight, C. Richard correctly understood that the clinical residency training experience that would be afforded to all would be vastly superior in a secular state-run setting in Newark.

It also gave the University of Medicine and Dentistry of New Jersey an affiliation with Beth Israel Hospital, a major cardiac center and venerable institution in the Jewish community since 1901 (referred to by Phillip Roth and others when talking about the varied cultural history of the Weequahic section of Newark where Beth Israel sits.) Of note, Mischa, my father, and I all wound up doing our internships there. One Sunday morning during my internship amid a bagels and cream cheese rounds, an elderly nurse when hearing my last name told me about looking out the window where we were then sitting and watching my father play basketball in the driveway of Mischa's house, which abutted the hospital grounds.

As it turned out, looking for medical school grads from around the world to bring to Newark also provided my father the opportunity to meet the owners of the schools in Cuernavaca and Grenada. This later was to prove more than helpful in my and my brother Marc's lives.

Not long after I married Ona (the mother of my daughter, Georgia), my father needed to have his aortic valve replaced and had it done at The Beth. This was in 1988, eight years after he had me listen to the murmur that informed me he was going to eventually have that procedure. He came out of the surgery a changed man, at least for a while. Suddenly, he was introspective. Instead of his usual glib responses to random questions, he'd now say, "What does that mean?" or "Why are you thinking about that?"

(Reading this now to my brother, Neil, and his wife, Andrea, Neil commented, "He softened, and he had 'heart' then.")

And while it didn't last for long, it was fascinating to see and to try to speculate on what had occurred during or after the surgery.

Before he reverted to his former self, he volunteered a story to us:

At dinner one night with my mother and Ona, he told us about the time when his own mother had had a major stroke and needed a tracheostomy. It was clear she would be on life support for the duration of her life. This was in 1959, and we had been in Europe then for an International Conference on Radiology being held in Munich. I was 11 years old and still remember how my father got a transatlantic call, and suddenly we were on the next flight back to the US. Clepe now related that, when he arrived at Beth Israel, he could see the dire, unsalvageable state that Anne was in. He left and returned shortly thereafter, bringing some morphine he had left over from the war. He went into her room and injected her with it, knowing it would stop her breathing and critically, end her suffering.

The three of us were all blown away as he'd never revealed that story from nearly thirty years before to anyone. I believe it was the (temporary) psychic change he'd undergone after open heart surgery that prompted him to reveal it to us that night.

CHAPTER 3

SYNCHRONICITY AND INSPIRED INSANITY

While my father was busy throughout his adult life with all his professional endeavors, my mother was pursuing a career as an artist that she'd begun in high school. (At a memorial service we had for her after her death at age 93, her remaining high school friends all remarked on how they'd always thought of her as the creative one among them). Starting when my brothers and I were adolescents, and over the next 40 years, she immersed herself in this endeavor, taking classes, producing work, and having shows throughout New Jersey and New York. She worked in collage, watercolor, sculpture, and construction, a la Joseph Cornell. Her knowledge of the art world was encyclopedic and when I was in high school, my parents also began acquiring an extensive collection of paintings, drawings, and sculptures. One piece was a Harry Bertoia chime that sat in the front foyer of our house and that adults, children, and grandchildren were never tired of ringing.

The house was filled with a constantly changing array of art from then on (that traveled later to Florida with them) that had a great influence on my own aesthetics. In fact, one of my fondest memories is the day that my mother and I met in the city to see the Picasso show at the Museum of Modern Art (MOMA) in the 80s. Walking through the exhibit with her, exchanging impressions and references, and seeing his work through each other's eyes, created a most wonderful afternoon of sharing.

Another great memory of her was when I was making a movie that Weissberg, and my dear friend and college roommate Donald Lipski, and I collaborated on in Madison. We needed to satisfy our science requirements to graduate and had, along with several of our friends, enrolled in a course aptly named Physics in the Arts. Weissberg, Donald, and I decided to make a movie about the newly recognized issue of water pollution. Our awareness of this had been brought into focus because recently, parts of Lake Erie had been seen spontaneously burning, flames leaping up from the surface of the lake due to the high concentration of petroleum-based contaminants in it.

We named the movie "Save Lake Erie (or still life with fruit)," and the (silent) film images showed various people, parched with thirst, running through different locations, trying to find unpolluted water to drink. I decided to enlist my mother to appear in it. She cameoed for several minutes, running through the woods, clutching her throat (and being knocked over at one point by our Samoyed, Rasputin, who'd decided to come along for the shoot).)

It was also around that time that I convinced my mother to get stoned (I knew my father wouldn't do it.) It was a beautiful summer afternoon, and we were in the backyard of the house in South Orange. I rolled up a joint, lit it and my mother cautiously, initially, and then with a bit more gusto, shared it with me. After a few minutes, I looked at her and asked if she felt anything.

She glanced back smiling and said, "I feel like the top of my head is coming off!"

With that, my father decided we had to go inside so he could put on "Give Me Shelter" from The Rolling Stones' album, *Beggars Banquet*. As soon as the music began, he started trying to see if he could cause any reactions from his now-stoned wife and son by making random noises and swirly hand and arm movements in front of our faces. When he got no particular response from us, he switched gears to talk about what he and his fellow World War II pilots sometimes did at high altitudes. He gave us a detailed description of how they would play around with the oxygen concentrations on their pressurized masks to see what kind of highs they could achieve.

Interestingly, I read several years ago how US and Nazi pilots used amphetamines to keep them going on their long, intense flights. My friend, Zeke, and I, at the age of 13 or so, found a Benzedrex inhaler of my father's that I'm sure dated back to wartime. We had no idea what it was, but I can still remember the smell and the buzz it gave us at the time.

By the end of college, things were starting to improve between my father and me, but earlier on, even before my adolescence, due to my own stubborn and determined nature, my father and I fought frequently. Whether about my grades (like Clepe, I was also a classic underachiever as a student), my clothes, or hair length, the dinner table was a frequent site of these jousts. Of course, it reached its culmination when I became outspoken in my opposition to the Vietnam War during my time in Madison.

Then his mantra became, "You should go into the Army. It'll make a man out of you." Only, behind the scenes, something else was playing out. He was sending me to a friend of his, a conservative shrink, every time I'd come home from college. This was ostensibly to "straighten me out".

I'd reluctantly go to the appointment, argue with this psychiatrist, tell him I planned to travel around Europe after college, and share other vague thoughts I had about my future. As I recall, he would tell me how unfocused and naive I was.

In the Fall of 1969, the first lottery for the draft took place. This was during the winter of my senior year at Madison, and unfortunately, I drew a low number. My draft physical was set for Monday, May 20, my 22nd birthday, in Newark. I flew home that weekend, shrink letter in hand from a psychiatrist we were all seeing in Madison. I hoped that his letter would get me a psychiatric 4-F classification, not eligible to serve. (At the same time, my mother's father, Jules, 79 and infirm, but a thoughtful, gentle man with very progressive leanings, had told me then that he wouldn't let me be "cannon fodder" and if I was drafted, he'd take me to Canada.)

That weekend, my parents, brothers, and I did our usual Sunday outing for Chinese food. On the way home, my father, seemingly randomly, stopped the car at the shrink's house and went inside. He didn't say a word to any of us, and I don't think anyone, but I knew whose house he was stopping in front of.

Fifteen minutes later, just as silently, my father reappeared, got back in the car, and we continued on our drive home. When we arrived, my mother and brothers went into the house, and my father, standing by the car, turned to me and said, "Kenny, I want to show you something."

With that, he pulled out, from its envelope, a three-page handwritten letter from the psychiatrist, on his official medical stationery.

I stood there and read it as my father watched.

What the psychiatrist had written was that I was manic depressive, a drug abuser, and homosexual, and had had an affair with one of my college professors!

None of it was true, and while the immediate import of what my father had done was apparent, it took me years to realize how meticulously he'd gone about orchestrating something that he knew would guarantee that I'd never serve a minute in the military.

I often, when I think of that scene, imagine my father standing behind the shrink, pointing a (figurative) gun to his head, and dictating exactly what he wanted written.

The next day, at the induction center in Newark, I met with the Army psychiatrist, tried to act depressed, and got a 1-Y classification. 1-Y was even more sketchy than 4-F, basically putting me in a category that said I'd only be eligible for the draft in case of a nuclear war. I also was the only one in the vast induction center walking around in jeans. Everyone else was in their boxers, but those days my friends and I were in a phase we called "hanging loose," not wearing underwear, and the draft officials quickly decided, after learning of my sartorial inclinations, that jeans were preferable to nude.

My father never intended for me to go in the Army or fight in a war I realized he was against as well. He had been sending me to the shrink, not really to "straighten me out" but to have a well-documented record of my having sought psychiatric care in case anyone got suspicious about my case.

Interestingly, as well, I suspect that my father's time in the Army Air Force, as it was then called, did help make a man out of him, as it did to so many of his generation. Being a flight surgeon, dealing with the dead, dying, and wounded in Europe (my father was stationed in The Azores, off the coast of Portugal,) I am sure put life in a very stark perspective. The other part of his response to serving in the war was that other than referring to a back injury he suffered when he was carrying a wounded man on a stretcher and the other person carrying dropped it, he never once talked to my brothers or me about what he saw during the time he served.

Because my father was such a dominant figure during my childhood, my mother was in certain ways in the background. Regardless, my brothers and I recognized that she was on our side, though, in most of the '60s and '70s battles that raged in our house. While she rarely, if ever, directly confronted our father amid the fights, Neil would tell me about the arguments she would have at night with him, defending me and my brothers, arguments that Neil would overhear through their closed bedroom door.

My mother, nevertheless, having grown up as that only child, protected daughter, had difficulty dealing with three growing, obstreperous boys. My brothers and I were all major belchers. This was not an uncommon calling among some of my peers as well. My friend David Levin could burp the entire Star-Spangled Banner on one forced inhale, and I believe that my own worsening reflux esophagitis was primed by my ventures deep into the realm of the belch. One evening, my mother and the three boys were sitting at the dinner table, having begun our evening meal before my father got back from work. My brothers and I were randomly exhibiting frequent eructatory outbursts in between bites of dinner, to my mother's chagrin.

Finally, in desperation, she said, "I just don't know where you boys got this from!"

Sure enough, as if on cue, at that moment my father opened the front door and let out a rather sonorous belch himself.

Not only did it answer my mother's question, but it put an end to the issue as well. And it was a good example of how my generally staid-appearing father was not so staid at all.

Interestingly, looking through my old journals, I came upon something I wrote around that time, feeling like my mother didn't love me because I never saw her stand up for me. I was shocked to read it, didn't remember that feeling at all, and knew it was clear where she was at in so many other ways. I remember frequently coming home at night from a basketball league I was part of in junior high and sitting with her in the kitchen talking about literature. She'd been an English lit major in college and had a love of books and a unique love of words, which she shared with us. She also had a subtle but wickedly ironic sense of humor that she imbued my brothers and me with as well.

When I was in college and started learning about the mysticism taught by Gurdjieff and Ouspensky, she recounted her own explorations of the work of Madame Blavatsky, co-founder of the Theosophical Society, a forerunner of the mystical teachings Gurdjieff espoused.

Also, my first exposure to the concepts of coincidence versus synchronicity is attributable to her. Early on, she told me a story about being at Beth Israel Hospital in Newark, ready to give birth to her first child (me). She didn't know if she was having a boy or a girl, but she and my father had decided that if it was a boy, he would be named Kenneth Robert. As she was lying in the delivery room, she was reading the Beth Israel Hospital Bulletin and saw an item that said that a son, Kenneth Robert, had just been born to Mr. and Mrs. Ned Weissberg of Elizabeth. Although my parents were living in Newark at the time, she thought, 'I wonder if we have a boy, if these two will ever meet and become friends.'

She delivered me, and five years later, we moved to South Orange, two blocks from where the Weissbergs had moved the year before. Weissberg and I met in kindergarten that year and have been best friends, and at times "worst enemies," for 70 years now. We grew up pushing limits of a verbal, intellectual, physical, and linguistic nature; getting in trouble; being kicked off Safety Patrol in 6th grade; going to the University of Wisconsin together and being put on social probation freshman year when we foolishly decided to become roommates. We developed a repertoire we call "Inspired Insanity" based on countless events, and bizarre personalities: the Czechoslovakian accent of my family's housekeeper, Mrs. Viparina; the French accent of my grandfather, Papa Jules Vaintrob; romantic foibles and successes; exotic references from across seven decades that either one of us can evoke in an instant with a text, phone call or deranged voicemail, bringing instant hilarity.

I believe our unique relationship has helped maintain my memory of a litany of events long past and more importantly, my sanity.

But was that reading by my mother a coincidence or synchronicity? Was my mother just paying attention, or was she plugged into things in ways that I think I am as well?

Not long after Ona and I met, we had a conversation about Jung and his concept of synchronicity. We decided to drive to Midtown and buy Jung's book, *Synchronicity*, at one of the many bookstores that still populated the area of Fifth Avenue in the mid-40s. We parked the car on East 39th Street and perused several of the stores on Fifth Avenue, including Rizzoli and Scribner's. None of them had the book. Disheartened, we went back to the car, only to find that we'd parked in front of the Jungian Institute. We walked in, bought *Synchronicity*, and returned home, marveling at what seemed a perfect example of the concept.

As I write this, it makes me wonder if I inherited my frequent experiences of synchronicity from my mother or merely learned her art of observation. In either case, perhaps it is why I've made so many strange connections over the years.

Finally, having lost my father in 2006, I find that his "Clepeisms" still pop up all the time: "It filled a void" to describe a meal that wasn't particularly tasty but got one over the hunger hump. Saying something is "Good for you, and it helps you too" for a nutritious if not necessarily scrumptious meal or medicine that quickly relieves one's symptoms.

Svigninabipkus (according to Clepe, "rabbit turds") for little meaningless items. And my last and favorite phrase: *es vet helfn vi a totynn bankes*. This Yiddish expression, meaning something is helpless, translates as "that is as helpful as putting cups on a dead person," cupping being a medical treatment of questionable validity.

My thoughts and memories of Renee, who died in 2017, are different and more subtle, often provoked by looking at her artwork, collages, and constructions that I have scattered throughout my house in Old Chatham and in New York City.

I see two sides of me, still exemplified by them: the aggressive, wisecracking, and at times, confrontational, Clepe, and the more reflective, ironic, and humble Renee. I am increasingly grateful for all that they passed on.

CHAPTER 4

WHILE READING *CITIES OF GLASS*

I attended The University of Wisconsin-Madison from 1966 through 1970. During my last two years there, I lived on a farm with three other guys of similar backgrounds. We all had met at the Jewish Fraternity, AEPi, and became fast friends. But as soon as The Revolution started in late 1967, and politics became increasingly important (and divisive with our more conventional fraternity brothers) we quickly left AEPi, downtown Madison, and moved out to the country. On our farm, along with two horses, interesting, abandoned outbuildings we explored and filmed, and a football field across the road lived my roommates: Eric Nathan from Manhattan, Donald Lipski from Highland Park, Illinois, and Rick Kleiner from Beverly Hills. We had similar backgrounds and appearances, so much so that we often were confused for one another when we were back on campus. But there was one major difference: While Donald's, Eric's, and my father were relatively conventional types, Rick's father, Burt, was an unconventional high roller. He headed a major brokerage firm on Rodeo Drive, as I recall, and had a beach house in Malibu. He was a wise guy with great stories and impressive friends in the film, literary, and art worlds. He was also a very generous man, giving money to many of the writers and struggling artists who came to him to get funding for their various projects. I was told by one of his friends, Benny Shapiro (who had run the British blockade of Palestine in 1948) that Burt would, in these situations ask how much money they needed, would give it to them, and then, almost as an afterthought, ask what they needed the money for. But it also allowed him to feel that he could borrow their interesting stories. Burt visited the farm one year for Rick's birthday and wound up taking LSD with us. At some point, he told us how he'd first gotten stoned, in 1954, with Louis Armstrong! It was a great story but turned out not to be true. I ran into Benny Shapiro years later in NYC and told him about Burt and Louis. He immediately said, "No! That happened to me. Burt liked that one so much that he appropriated it." In any case, Donald and I (maybe not so much Eric) were a bit jealous of Rick. Not only was he living on the farm with one of Madison's most intriguing beauties, but he also had his artsy, hipster father and all that Burt's lifestyle, wealth, and influential friends had to offer.

In those days, it was largely for the good: When my interest in Jewish mysticism was piqued, I went to see Rabbi Herbert Weiner, the man who'd bar mitzvahed me (and later performed the marriage ceremony for me and my first wife, Lois). I'd learned from Clepe and Renee that the rabbi had a deep involvement in the world of Kabbalah, the Jewish mystical teachings. I met with him and found out he'd written a book, *The Wild Goats of Ein Gedi*, about his travels in Israel and meeting Jewish holy men there. I mentioned *The Wild Goats* to Rick, and because he and Burt had a connection with Alan Watts, the well-known popularizer of mysticism, they introduced Weiner and Watts. As I mention in the story, "On Succos Reciting the Bruchas", the rabbi's book sales took off as Watts frequently referred to it as he spoke around the country. And years later, when I'd already become a doctor, I was in San Francisco and met with another connection of Burt's, Dr. Stanley Krippner. Krippner is a psychologist studying dream states and the paranormal, and interestingly, when I met him, he was the Alan Watts Professor of Psychology at Saybrook University in Oakland. Stanley and I had a great conversation, and I bought and read his book, *The Realms of Healing*. These connections were very exciting to take advantage of, but, as the years went by, we began to realize that the relationship of Rick and Burt was starting to evolve into what would become a disturbing and deadly cautionary tale.

In Madison the protests got worse; we were initiated into the smell of tear gas and how to mitigate its effects; some of us got arrested and hurt, as we lived through the crescendo of outrage over Vietnam and the draft; the protests that culminated in the killings of students at Mississippi State and Kent State and the death of a graduate student when the Army Math Research Center was blown up in Madison in the summer of 1970. I only graduated because the country was in such turmoil in the Spring of '70 that all classes at UW became Pass/Fail, and I was able to receive my BA, barely, in TV and Film Production. Rick Kleiner chose not to graduate. In the Spring of 1970, through Burts connections, he was offered a job working on a film with the avant-garde filmmaker Alejandro Jodorowsky in Mexico. He packed up his van and left Madison, never staying around the extra two months he would have needed to get his degree.

A year or so later, back in NYC, I had that brief, too-early marriage presided over by Rabbi Weiner. It was a wedding that my parents refused to attend, thinking we were too young. When the marriage ended in 1974 (my parents' non-acceptance of it hadn't helped) I moved into a loft at 6 Varick Street, in the area that came to be known as Tribeca. I lived on the top floor of a great cast iron building at the corners of West Broadway, Varick, and Franklin Streets.

While I was alone on the 10th floor at night, during the day, I was engulfed by the smells of vanilla from my neighboring loft, a company that wholesaled vanilla extract called *Arominilla*, and enjoyed the camaraderie of the Pomponio Brothers. They were the owners of a machine shop on the floor, and they befriended me when I moved in after I gave them an ugly barcalounger that had been left in my loft. Very generous men, they let me use their tools as I renovated my space, installing a darkroom and a claw leg tub in the kitchen. It was a very exciting time, I was on my own as a young adult, and I was desperately trying to figure out how to pursue a career in film. Kleiner actually moved in with me for a while there, but his downward turn had already begun. I had to kick him out after I learned that not only was he stealing from me, but because my toilet was out in the hall, too much of a nuisance for him to access, he decided that he could just aim his dick through my window and pee down into the street. He later showed up at Eric's apartment and pulled a similar number: stealing from him as well, though not the rest, as Eric did have an en-face bathroom in his more traditional place.

And in the crazy way of the world, years later after my career path had changed and I'd become a practicing ER doc, I was reading my first Paul Auster novel, *Cities of Glass*. I discovered that he too had clearly lived on my floor at 6 Varick. His book was set there, and in it, he talked about the Pomponios. I wrote him a letter, through his publisher, and told him that, though his novels seemed to always be set a few degrees from reality, he clearly couldn't have made up those brothers. I realized he must have lived on the 10th floor not long after me, two South Orange Boys holing up in the wilds of downtown Manhattan in the '70s. He wrote back and told me how my letter had arrived, "like manna from heaven," we established a loose relationship after that, including him referencing a Dr. Weinberg character in one of his subsequent books.

Back to 6 Varick. I was freelancing in film, working in the darkroom, and exploring what I could do with the very first portable video equipment ever available, rented from a place 3 blocks south of my loft on West Broadway. I started working on a piece I hoped to sell to Sterling Manhattan Cable on the uses people were making of the partly dismantled West Side Highway. It had just been abandoned to traffic when an overloaded truck crashed through a section on Gansevoort Street.

It was a hard yet reflective time, a lot of hustling, trying to pay the rent and have a career in film. As fate would have it, I started working on more and more medically oriented-films and tapes.

Just before I moved from Brooklyn, one of my closest, brilliant friends, Robby Grossman, moved in. I'd known him since high school, and he'd been an influence in my decision to enroll in college at the University of Wisconsin. Robby had been drifting for a while in Madison and thereafter. This was not a difficult or unusual thing to do in the late '60s/ early '70s with the draft, protests against Dow Chemical Corporation and the Vietnam War, Be-ins and sex, drugs, and rock n' roll affecting all of us so deeply.

Now, a few years later, Robby was back on track. He'd decided to go to medical school and had just finished his first year in the Philippines. He needed somewhere to stay as he studied for Part 1 of the National Medical Boards, and he moved into the apartment.

Robby hated the Philippines and hoped to do well enough on the boards to transfer back to an American school. He scored possibly the highest in the world on the boards and was accepted into med school at Albert Einstein that year. He subsequently went on to a distinguished career as an interventional cardiologist and later, an elected public health official in Los Angeles.

While he was staying with me, I started reading Robby's medical texts and found them very approachable and extremely interesting, although they also gave me a sense of the enormity of what there was to learn and understand as a physician.

Now, alone in my loft, with time for reflection and months of consideration, I had an epiphany that put everything in perspective: "If Robby can become a doctor, so can I."

I had also realized that I was not a pushy go-getter and lacked internal discipline, two things a freelance film person needed to be and have. I decided that if I went to medical school, its external discipline would force me to study and that if I kept things together, in four years or so, I'd become a doctor.

It also became increasingly clear that I could be creative as a physician, pursuing the interactions between mind and body that even as a child I'd had floating around in my brain.

During this time, my youngest brother Marc came to live with me. He'd graduated from New College in Sarasota the year before and was trying to figure out what to do with his life. We spent a lot of time that year talking and grappling with the issue of whether we could successfully follow in the Weinberg family tradition (having grown up being frequently asked if we were going to be "the next Dr. Weinberg.") Soon he too decided that he would pursue medicine and after we finished shooting the West Side Highway video together, we enrolled in the School of General Studies at Columbia to take our unfinished premed courses.

Luckily for me, I was able to opt out of physics because of my two semesters of "Physics for Poets". This had been the fabulous, hands-on lab course for which I shot the film, "Save Lake Erie". The course was taught by two brilliant Madison physics professors. My friends and I all assumed, correctly

I think, that they had decided to run the classes so they could sleep with the radical hippie chicks. Be that as it may, it now allowed me to opt out of the medical school physics requirement.

A year later, Marc and I found ourselves studying in Guadalajara, Mexico, or as my dear friend, Eric Nathan, upon visiting us there, called it: "God, What a Horror."

CHAPTER 5

LITTLE MAN SYNDROME

"Oh my god! Look at those fucking cadavers floating in the brine."

Marc and I were starting our first semester in Guad. And we had just learned that, before we could ever enter the Anatomy Lab, each incoming student had to procure one of these corpses. The bodies were barely visible, obviously dumped randomly, one atop another, in a deep, concrete-lined vat, reeking of formaldehyde. After we managed to pull them out of this foul-smelling swill, we'd be using them for our dissections over the next 6 months. And we were told rather matter-of-factly that these bodies we were going to be working on were not deceased Mexicans but Haitians.

It didn't take too long to figure out the reason for that. We had started med school in 1977, in the days of the right-wing Duvalier regime in Haiti. Among its many atrocities, this regime was an early adopter of the policy of "disappearing" its enemies. We knew that our medical school, the Universidad Autonoma de Guadalajara, or UAG, had been started by a group of hard-right upper-class Mexicans. They started it in opposition to the state medical school, long known for its left-wing politics. And it didn't take a leap of brilliance to understand that there probably was no more convenient place to dispose of "disappeareds" from Haiti than into the anatomy vats of a school in Mexico, whose political persuasions lined up with those of Papa and Baby Doc Duvalier.

Our next lesson in the macabre ways of medical education in Mexico came when we were told that we should all buy a skeleton to keep at home to be able to visualize and understand the relationships of the bones in the human body. The second-year American students, who'd taken us under their wings, said we needed to go to the local cemetery, and there we would be able to purchase these bones. We were advised, though, to make sure to get them "con calcetinas", with socks, if we wanted to get a complete skeleton, not one missing the feet.

Marc, whose sense of humor and irony was always just below the surface, found this tremendously amusing, and soon, con calcetinas entered our lexicon in an evolving variety of situations.

These early introductions began to alert us to some of the unique customs of the UAG and Guadalajara and what we might expect during our hopefully brief sojourn there (like almost every American enrolled in medical school anywhere abroad, we intended to focus intently on studying for and passing Part 1 of the National Medical Boards so we could transfer back to a US school after two years).

And who were we medical gringoes? A diverse and mostly reasonable group of overly well-qualified Americans who had been trying for years to get into a U.S. med school and finally, despite a master's degree in biology, PhDs in physiology, careers in allied medical fields from medic to undertaker, had thrown in the towel and headed outside the country.

My brother, Marc, and I, on the other hand, were outliers in this group, in that we hadn't even tried to get into American schools, our unique and undistinguished college resumes being what they were.

When I'd been in Madison I'd been living on the farm, getting involved with Students for a Democratic Society, and deciding after my first semester as a pre-med that 7:45 a.m. chemistry lectures were not going to happen. With The Revolution going on, Be-ins, acid trips, and an anarchic lifestyle, what seemed much more compelling and reasonable were creative pursuits. I decided that I'd rather be an artist than a physician and opted to follow in the footsteps of my mother. Being the youngest of three brothers, I don't remember Marc having quite the same pressure, or influence from my father or grandfather that I did to go into medicine. (I do remember my grandfather coming to our house with large cardboard sheets he'd covered with copious handwritten notes in his Cyrillic style, about all the blood groups. His last years in medicine were spent as the Attending Physician at the Garden State Blood Bank in Newark). He sat with me for several hours to teach me about Groups A, B, AB and O, and Rh factor when I was in ninth grade. I even did a science project where I pricked my friends' fingers or knees to get blood and identify what their blood type was. Marc, being five years younger, never had this type of interaction with Mischa.

It's interesting for me to think about the fact that none of the three brothers ever really talked among ourselves about following in the footsteps of our father or grandfather while we were growing up. Our grandfather was too distant in our lives and when we all still lived together, our very close relationship was largely based on, and created by, our opposition to our father and his intrusive, overbearing ways.

Back to God, What a Horror. We also had our share of offbeat colleagues in the Guad, to say the least. Shiptalk and Pyramid Mike were two of the more not diverse but more like divergent of them.

"Shiptalk", as we surreptitiously named him because of his constant use of military jargon, had some kind of checkered past as a medic in the Navy, as I recall. Little Man Syndrome, nasty and paranoid, with phrases acquired and honed over years in God knows what medical trenches. I remember his talking about the pleasure he got in resuscitating trauma victims by placing huge 14-gauge IV catheters ("large enough to read the NYT through") in their forearms. And despite the bonding and the camaraderie all of the American students felt for one another, I most remember him for one day threatening to spill the beans on us.

I can't recall exactly what triggered the sudden confrontation he had with us that time between classes, but I do know it was in response to one of our many subversive attempts to dance around the school's heinous, autocratic rules aimed at the despised, overeducated gringoes. Maybe it was comments we made about the histology professor, head of the Mexican Fascist Party, pistol always evident, tucked just inside his suit jacket, who made a point to come up to each of us as we labored over our microscopes to tell us, "Be careful, we are watching you."

Or perhaps it was about the surreptitious way we attempted to communicate with one another during our exams, tests written using obscure Spanish idioms designed to trick non-native speakers into answering the opposite way they intended. Whatever had caused it, we soon discovered, to our chagrin, that Shiptalk was a Tecolote (owl), or spy for UAG, a position that gave him tremendous leverage over the rest of us. As I think about it, I recall it was our use of the "Foot System" that triggered the conflict. This was something passed on to us by the older, more seasoned, and cynical second and third-year students.

At exam time, all the American students would attempt to sit next to one another in the same rows. When most of us were done with the test, someone would clear their throat. This was the signal to collectively and surreptitiously check our answers. While we'd all put our heads down as if reviewing our own exams, we would actually be using our peripheral vision to look at the outstretched feet of our neighbors. We would methodically go through the answers with each of us putting forward right foot for answer "A," right foot back "B," left foot forward "C," back "D," both forward "E," back "F."

Crossed feet indicated "I haven't a clue." And while this altercation with Shiptalk fortunately only caused a minor kerfuffle for a few of us, it led to our immediate and total alienation from him.

Then there was Pyramid Mike, a nice enough redheaded, Italian guy from Westchester County, NY. Before entering med school, he'd become convinced that placing anything under a pyramidal structure created tremendous healing energy, whether it be resharpening dull razor blades or curing cancer. He made many allusions to the Great Pyramids, their secrets, and their ability to preserve anything inside them.

He let us know that he slept under a pyramid set up over his bed and while the UAG rules prohibited students from having hair that reached below the collar, mustaches extending below the lips, or flip-flops in class, Mike was allowed to roam the campus wearing a pyramid on his head made of eight thin copper tubes. No one in charge even blinked an eye, though most of the gang that I hung out with, open-minded as we might be, were a bit nonplussed by it all.

I think the fact that Marc and I were there together helped save our sanity in this disturbing environment. We were not used to stooges and abject different rules for different people. Fortunately, we were there together and quickly realized what we'd have to do to stay under the radar and get out of Guad as quickly as possible.

We also were saved by the fact that the two of us rented a house in a nice, comfortable middle-class area of Guadalajara. It had an upstairs room that Marc eventually made his bedroom.

We quickly equipped the large living room with a ping-pong table. (This was a reprise of what we'd grown up with, a ping pong table in the basement. My father was a wicked opponent, with an ever-changing repertoire of spins, backhands, slices, and feints, accompanied by a repartee he'd acquired during his undergraduate time in Chapel Hill. My mother, on the other hand, had very strict rules when she deigned to take her turn with the paddle. "Boys, remember. No spins, no slams!")

When we needed a break in Guad, we would play Benny Goodman loudly on the cassette deck and have table tennis marathons between us and our friends. Our parents came to visit that first year, as well, and my father took great pleasure in bringing us his old med school textbooks and bonding with us, teaching and quizzing us on anatomy. I have a warm image of my mother sitting in the living room doing drawings of the Mexican landscape while Marc, my father, and I sat at our round, leather-covered Mexican table, and my father went through his wonderful Frank Netter illustrated books on various disease states, interspersed with his recollections of pre-med anatomy classes, working on cadavers with his older brother Arthur.

Other strategies we used to break up the craziness, especially that engendered by studying medicine in Spanish for UAG and in English to pass the boards, were frisbee extravaganzas with friends on the large open field by our house, horseback riding, and when we could, going to the beautiful and isolated beach in San Blas, in the state of Nayarit, for its amazing bird watching and many miles of long body-surfing cove. This all helped us endure the lunacy in class. For some reason, one of the professors, during the mandatory daily roll call, wound up calling one of us

Wineburg and the other Weenburg-we never knew who was who—and being forced each semester for two weeks to drive two hours out of town each day on the Guardia (literally guarding) to allegedly bring medical help to the impoverished peasants in their towns. In another one of the cruel ironies of UAG, we would take their medical histories, examine them as best we could, and then prescribe medicines to these innocent, indigent campesinos, prescriptions that everyone at the school knew few would be able to afford. We discovered that the "care" we were compelled to provide them was not due to the kindness of the owners of the med school but because that had been the only way the state of Jalisco would allow a second medical school to exist in Guadalajara alongside the government-run facility.

Guad was so bad that Clepe offered us an alternative. Calling in his chits for all the FMG (foreign med school grads) he had taken into the Newark City Hospital residencies, he approached the head of a med school in Cuernavaca he'd been dealing with. Guillermo, who had established the school several years before, was able and happy to accommodate what became a small exodus of Guad students.

Marc, me, my girlfriend Helene, and several of our friends wound up transferring to his school, Centro de Estudios Universitarios Xochicalco. The doctors were true clinicians, were people we could really respect and learn from, had much better politics, and Cuernavaca was a lovely town to live in. One of my most notable memories from that time was accompanying Dr. Naranjo, our pulmonary professor, to one of the indigent ERs in Mexico City one night. Naranjo supervised the ER, and I'll never forget an elderly patient he treated then who came in with congestive heart failure. His heart's pumping ability was severely compromised. It couldn't pump out all the blood coming back into it, and his lungs were filling up. The treatment that was employed, "rotating tourniquets," had been in use for at least fifty years before that, but we knew that, had this man come into a hospital in the United States, no one would have been placing painful, constricting bands on his upper thighs and arms to minimize the volume of blood coming back to his heart. This was el barrio in Mexico City in 1978, and clearly, no other form of treatment was available.

Despite the stress of living in a foreign country, learning about medicine in two languages, and living with the uncertainty of what the future would hold, after two years for Marc and three years for me, we were able to leave Mexico behind and dive into clinical rotations back in the States. We took with us the residue of very frightening and wonderful experiences: On one Guardia Marc and his friends spent a night in a Mexican jail, incarcerated and released at the whim of two Jefes (police chiefs) in a small town outside Guad. Another time, our brother Neil came to visit, and the three of us were stopped by 20-year-old machine gun-toting Federales, late at night on the way to a weekend in San Blas. Trying to be nonchalant, we stood outside the car as the soldiers spent what felt like hours searching our car (unsuccessfully) for any remnants of the marijuana they rightly suspected we'd been using.

Fortunately, as well, we had the forging of long-lasting friendships with several of our med school compatriots and a very satisfying love of and facility in the Spanish language.

That stands me in good stead to this day in so many situations, both medical and cultural.

After a torturous and circuitous four years, I finally finished med school, getting my degree from St. George's University in Grenada (the school in Cuernavaca, it turned out, was one of two schools with the same name and after a flurry of attempts, including meeting with the Governor of the State of Morelos to determine our school's legitimacy, I was able to transfer my credits to St. George's, another one of Clepe's chits.) But this unorthodox entry into the medical field was to be played out my whole career as I never uncloaked myself totally from the "outlier" status and pursued a career that was not the typical trajectory of a private practice doctor. I went more into unexpected and maybe challenging places. Guad was just the beginning of it.

CHAPTER 6

RED BLANKET ROOM

Prior to graduating from St. George's, I had to apply through the Match Program to various residencies and more importantly, I had to decide in what field I should do my training. I was torn between going into Internal Medicine or Psychiatry. For as long as I could remember, long before college, I'd always believed that the brain could affect how the body responded to various disease states. I think that this feels like something I intuited from time spent with my grandfather, Mischa, as well as my father, whose attitudes about most illnesses seemed to be to ignore, not focus on them, and they'd go away. And they usually would.

I ultimately decided that getting a deep understanding of the workings of the body would always stand me in good stead, so I opted to do an Internal Medicine residency.

I was accepted (one of three Foreign Medical School grads out of 32 incoming Interns) into, and began, at the University of Medicine and Dentistry of New Jersey (UMDNJ) in Newark. This was July 1, 1980.

Just before I was to start my internship, we had a family dinner. My father presented me with a Littman cardiology stethoscope, a special graduation gift. With my mother and two brothers sitting at the dining room table, he said, as I took the valued, prestigious scope from its box, "Kenny, listen to my heart."

I put in the two earpieces and placed the bell on his chest.

"Dad, you have a murmur!"

It was the murmur of aortic stenosis.

He nodded his head in agreement and nothing more was said. We all found out later that this was his way of telling us about the abnormal aortic valve he'd been born with and that, within a few years, would require him, at the age of 63, and then again at 86, to undergo cardiac surgery to have it replaced.

Finally feeling I was now more in the mainstream of medicine, I began my internship in Newark at the hospital where my father had been the director not too many years before.

A few things, of many, stand out about that year: the residency director was a hematologist ironically named Dr. Klotz, and for one month, my brother Marc was my medical student there. (He'd been accepted into UMDNJ med school on the proviso that he'd redo his second year, so I'd leaped ahead of him). As he reminded me at my 50th birthday celebration, it was that year 1980/81 that he and I saw our first AIDS patient together.

After several months in Newark, I had vacation time, and I went out to visit Robby, now Doctor Grossman, who was doing a Cardiology Fellowship at UCLA. While staying at his house in Westwood, I met and started to fall in love with Robby's girlfriend's sister. (Robby was now in a relationship with Rick Kleiner's former Madison girlfriend). After I returned East, the long-distance relationship blossomed, and I decided to transfer my residency to Los Angeles. I chose LA County Hospital, and with Dr. Klotz and other docs' letters of recommendation, I was accepted into my second year there. It was a great decision, even though my new girlfriend dumped me almost as soon as I arrived in Santa Monica, to start the residency. But I did have my Madison buddies, Rick Kleiner and of course, Robby, with whom I spent a lot of time in our new incarnation as doctors.

Rick, early on, asked me to do a house call on Burt. I found him, 15 years or so since I'd taken that acid trip with him in Madison, in terrible shape. He'd gotten addicted to narcotics and had developed COPD and a bizarre, obscure neurologic condition. I did what I could for Burt and saw Rick from time to time while I lived in LA. Not long after I saw Burt, Rick wound up moving in with him in Beverly Canyon. As I didn't stay in touch much, I didn't realize that Rick was continuing down what would turn out to be a deadly path.

LA County/USC turned out to be an excellent place to train (of note though, when I started there in July of 1981, the USC residency director read me the letter from Dr Klotz. While he had been very positive in his recommendation, he'd also apparently felt compelled to say of my interest in the mind/body interactions: that it was well-meaning, but "naïve.")

USC was run by brilliant, dedicated academic Attending Physicians in charge of the various departments; the patient mix was incredibly diverse (and often overwhelmingly ill); and as opposed to some academic institutions where there was a lot of handholding, at USC the house staff (interns, residents and fellows) ran the show. We were there all day (and frequently night) managing, treating patients, and learning in real-time how our decisions affected the outcomes of these patients (generally for good but sometimes not.) I came to understand how important this type of learning environment is for building the self-confidence (sans arrogance) that is vital to allow any of us to be competent, confident practitioners.

It was also there that I developed a love for the writing of Charles Bukowski, who lived in L.A. I saw him in so many of the down and out-patients we had to deal with, the ones we'd be called to see in the Red Blanket Room. This was the critical care area where the sickest patients would come from the Emergency Room to be admitted by those of us on call for the Internal Medicine team.

One version of Bukowski I will never forget was Mr. S., a longtime alcoholic, whom I cared for when I was rotating through six weeks in the Hepatology (Liver) service. It was a much sought-after rotation, taught by the brilliant Liver Specialist, Telfer Reynolds. Telfer was a stately, patrician doctor, with a shock of wavy, white hair, and when he first introduced me to Mr. S., it was clear he'd dealt with him many times before.

We'd come upon this patient in the Red Blanket Room, his face enclosed by a Blakemore-Sengshausen tube. At that time, it was pretty much the only treatment we had for patients who were bleeding from ruptured veins in the esophagus. The "tube" is a sturdy, round metal device, straddling the nose and mouth. It is attached to a long rubber hose with a big balloon at the far end. This balloon passes into the upper stomach and is then pulled tight. The tightness on the balloon end of this contraption is intended to put pressure on the bleeding veins in the esophagus and resembles a medieval torture instrument with its two metal halos, one above the other, pushing into the face. Yet even through, or perhaps because of, this contraption, Mr. S. was able to somewhat articulately curse out Dr. Reynolds as the doctor calmly and respectfully attempted to obtain the history of his present admission.

As I was finishing my third year and considering my next move, I had several options I was thinking about: One of the LA County internists offered me a job in his office, and I was considering a fellowship in Rheumatology or Infectious Disease. But when I pursued these latter two options, I was told that because I was an FMG, the trajectory of my career in academic medicine would not go very far. I also began corresponding with Dr. John Rotrosen. I had done research as a medical student with John, who'd been in a psychiatry residency at NYU when we found each other living at 6 Varick Street (John and I'd known each other years before from Columbia High School). He'd subsequently become the chair of the Psychiatry Department at the Manhattan VA (part of NYU), and we'd stayed in touch during my residency.

John and I began having extensive conversations about my moving back to NYC and working under him. I was interested in fashioning my own Fellowship at the VA in an area that was just starting to emerge in Mind/body medicine called Psychoneuroimmunology.

The fellowship we started to discuss was a very exciting proposition that would allow me to pursue my interests even, especially when, they went into controversial areas. I'd be doing this in a state-of-the-art research department affiliated with a major medical center. I felt myself moving towards this option because anytime I discussed alternative medical treatments with my colleagues or attending physicians, they always dismissed any positive findings as "purely anecdotal". I felt like this fellowship at a strongly research-oriented facility would allow me to do well-designed studies whose results, if positive, could not be so easily dismissed.

As the residency ended, I felt great about the arrangement John and I were making, and I eagerly agreed to move back to New York. However, the day before I was to leave, I had a disturbing event with Robby and Rick. Rick had asked if he could drive back to NYC with me. He was at my apartment when Robby showed up to wish me goodbye. Rick left soon thereafter, and Robby immediately turned to me and said, "Kenny, you are nuts if you intend to drive back with Kleiner! Can't you see how fucked up he is? His drug issue is out of control, and I really believe it would be dangerous for you to make the drive cross country with him." At his insistence (I hate telling people things that might make them angry with me), I called Rick and canceled the drive, arranged for the car to be transported to NY, and flew back there myself.

Not long after this event, the drug dealer supplying both Rick and Burt confronted Rick at the home he and Burt were living in in Beverly Canyon. Rick apparently owed him a lot of money and the man came at Rick with a knife. The story we were all told was that Rick grabbed the knife away and stabbed the dealer twenty-eight times, killing him.

Fortunately for Rick, because of family connections, he was convicted of manslaughter, not murder, and spent the next four years in the penitentiary on Terminal Island.

I've thought about this turn of events many times and come to realize that maybe having a "cool" father wasn't so great after all. It made me appreciate Clepe and his steadiness a lot more and gave me pause when my daughter was born, several years later. I realized I needed to be more aware of the boundaries I might have otherwise pushed with her and her friends when she became an adolescent. Ultimately, Burt Kleiner was not a father figure to emulate.

My acceptance letter from the head of NYU's Psychiatry Department was notable, I thought. In addition to being very happy to have me join the department, he wrote that he hoped I'd "have a lot of fun."

Fun it was! The Manhattan VA Psychiatry Department Rotrosen ran was very collaborative and filled with smart, and not surprisingly, limit-pushing types. One was Burt

Angrist, a prodigiously published researcher in the field of schizophrenia, who also was a member of The Vulgarians. Loosely begun in the 1950s, they were a group of scientists and physicians who went rock climbing (often in the nude and after having ingested psychedelics) in the "Gunks", a beautiful mountain ridge in New Paltz, New York.

One day, Burt and I volunteered for a study on the effects of intravenous apomorphine (a dopamine-type drug that was being looked at for a better understanding of neurotransmitters, a newly burgeoning field). We sat in a small room where we each were to have an IV placed, after which we would receive increasingly high aliquots of the drug. As the dose increased, we were to describe our physical and mental reactions to a medical transcriptionist. As Burt sat, right arm extended, tourniquet in place, and IV line at the ready, he began to recite a line to me from William Burroughs's *Naked Lunch.* It was one of many in the book describing Burroughs and his friends' experience of shooting drugs.

"The red rose of blood blossomed in the dropper..."

I was a Burroughs aficionado, and at that moment laughed uproariously and understood, not surprisingly, that Burt was as well.

Another person affiliated with the group was Dr. Arnold Lippa, Ph.D. He'd drive in from Sandoz Laboratories to give lectures on his work in the field of neurotransmitters. Lippa was a brilliant and provocative neuroscientist looking at, among other things, the study of *dysphorilytics* (drugs that lyse or break up dysphoria, a profound state of unease.)

As the year began, I was treating psych patients, vets who'd wound up in the locked ward at the VA, including one who became my favorite patient, Franklin S. Franklin had been assaultive and aggressive when he was admitted, but by the time I began taking care of him, he was pleasant and interactive, though still delusional. Among his many benignly delusional references, he decided to call me his "Nautical man". Ona, my soon-to-be wife, upon hearing this, wrote me a poem, dedicated to "Her Nautical Man".

After a year or more, Franklin, no longer delusional, finally seemed ready to qualify for an outpatient facility. We brought him to one in Brooklyn, he took the tour, met several of the other residents and when we asked him what he thought of them, his response was, "I don't know but it seems like a number of these guys are a bit *mishuqee*."

In addition to treating my own patients, I was also working with the liaison psychiatry team seeing medical patients with psychiatric issues and interacting with the brilliant and provocative Dr. Mack Lipkin, who'd begun (and still runs) the Primary Care Department at NYU.

It was New York in the early 80s and a very exciting time. At night, I'd often join friends at the Great Jones Cafe, a raucous downtown restaurant and bar, for meals and late-night drunken poetry readings. For a few brief moments, I hung out there with filmmaker Paula L. Paula (who among her many other claims to fame had the distinction of being the only person I knew who had hot and cold running water in the toilets of her Tribeca loft) was tickled at having met, as she said, "a conceptual doctor." One day during our abbreviated but spicy romance, she presented me with a wonderful T-shirt she'd inscribed with images of various bugs, bacteria, and medical devices to illustrate what she imagined my research was all about.

Soon, working with Dr. Wafaa El-Sadr, an infectious disease physician (who not long thereafter would become world famous for her work on HIV), we decided to do a study to look at the effects of acupuncture on AIDS patients. We hoped this treatment might stimulate their malfunctioning immune systems. AIDS was still a very newly discovered and little-understood, disease entity then, and there were no treatments yet available at the time. I spent seven months on this study, including learning how to work in an immunology lab to demonstrate if acupuncture might have a measurable effect on T cells.

After seven months, my AIDS/acupuncture project was finally approved by the Human Subjects Committee, and I went to sign up my first patients. It was 1984, and every one of them was thrilled to enter the study since being given a diagnosis of AIDS was then a death sentence. We intended to use sterile, non-reusable acupuncture needles and had found two very qualified acupuncturists who'd be doing the treatment. I'd be looking in the lab to see if there was any improvement in their T-cell function during and after the acupuncture.

Wafaa was in China when the study was slated to begin, but her colleague, Michael Simberkoff, who was also treating AIDS patients at the VA, was on the wards when I was enrolling patients. Simberkoff got wind of what was happening and was outraged that we were going to be treating "his" AIDS patients with acupuncture.

I was soon called into the office of Dr. Nortie Spritz, the head of the Department of Medicine. Spritz acted as if he had known nothing of the study until he'd been alerted by Simberkoff (even though Dr. Spritz was on the Human Subjects Committee that had finally approved it). Spritz told me he wouldn't allow the study to proceed and when I asked why, was told it was because he didn't "want the VA to be known as a place that practiced Voodoo Medicine."

I was aghast and went back to Rotrosen, who ducked. His surprising response made me hurt and angry and caused me to quickly realize I could no longer stay in the Fellowship.

When I told John I was quitting, he told me that he'd learned, "a long time ago not to fight battles I can't win."

I wished I had known that before I'd started the Fellowship, as I'd made it clear that I was going to be looking at controversial issues. I had only returned to New York as I had assumed John would have my back.

Now here I was, in New York, about to get married, and I needed a job.

CHAPTER 7

God Bless Bellevue

Dr. Sara W., a friend, was very sympathetic to my plight and wondered, based on my moonlighting experiences in the ER at the VA and LA County, how I'd feel about working in an Emergency Department until I figured things out.

Sara and I had met when she was studying psychiatry at NYU (also like me, after doing an Internal Medicine residency) and dated for a while. It turned out also that she'd, like my brother Neil, been in the first class at the newly opened Hampshire College in Amherst, Massachusetts in 1970.

I hadn't really considered Emergency Medicine at that point. In fact, during my residency in Internal Medicine at Los Angeles County, we scorned the ER docs. Called them "cowboys." (Of course, they called us "fleas" because, to them, we focused on irrelevant minutia.) And it was common amongst my Internal Medicine colleagues to disdainfully recount how often the patients we got from the ER wound up being so different than what they were billed to us when we were called in to admit them by our Emergency Medicine compatriots.

But I did need a job, so Sara suggested I contact Dr. Lewis Goldfrank, the Director of the NYU and Bellevue Emergency Departments. I applied for the job and after interviewing with Lewis, got hired.

That began a friendship with Lewis that lasts to this day. The Emergency Department was well run and staffed by very dedicated MDs, nurses, and Nurse Practitioners. I soon realized Goldfrank was a mensch, and it was because of him and the other practitioners at Bellevue that I developed a great understanding of, and respect for, the newly emerging specialty of Emergency Medicine. And I wound up ultimately, becoming board certified in the field.

Bellevue was also where I first started formally writing. Lewis recognized my medical abilities, my literary interests, and my moral/philosophical concerns as well. He started passing along assignments writing for a Physician Assistant magazine on medical ethics, which I eagerly took on. I was also able to publish my first case study, on a patient I'd treated with cardiac Munchausen's Syndrome (this man was so good at appearing to be having a heart attack that, when in the ICU, he'd learned how to manipulate the electrical leads on his chest to make it look on the cardiac monitor that he was experiencing ventricular fibrillation). This was also when, deep into several particularly crazy shifts, I also came to find myself thinking of literary and cinematic motifs in the patient encounters I was having. Doing this, being reminded of scenes from Marx Brothers movies or lines from, for example, Catch-22 amused me and gave me a different, healthier perspective on what I was so caught up in at that moment.

The work at Bellevue was exciting and intellectually challenging, and the emergency physician lifestyle provided a freedom that suited me and appealed to my dislike of routine.

I wound up, through this kind of doctoring, becoming aware, and increasingly appreciative, that I'd become a very astute, competent physician, getting to deeply know about every bodily system and how they interacted, being acutely cued into how dysfunction in one bodily part sometimes mimicked another part's symptoms and teasing that out so I could quickly and successfully intervene.

I loved that, as an ER doctor, I could jump in and fix the medical problem or do a good quick stabilization in those situations when something terrible had just occurred. These situations not infrequently occur, not just at work, but also on the tennis court, on an airplane, or anywhere the call, "Is there a doctor available?" go out.

It was also at Bellevue that I started writing stories. It's not easy to imagine (although people always ask) the array of patients and their dramas that I was exposed to there, and I felt the need to jot down my interactions and impressions.

I would come home after my shifts often carrying written "snippets" of an event that had just occurred and once I'd slept a bit, write a story of the incredible comedie humaine (and tragique) that had transpired. Over the years, I wrote about thirty of these stories. They were about those ephemeral moments that doctors and nurses on the front lines experience: the moment before, and the moment after, when everything changes irrevocably in patients' and their families' lives. The moments when all artifice is ripped away, frankly because the patient or family member is scared out of their mind about the imminent loss of life or limb or autonomy. The narratives described how we, as practitioners, have a few fraught instants in those encounters to turn things around, or sometimes not.

My writing not only tried to capture those occasions but also, I've come to understand, provided an effective and healthy coping mechanism through my forty-year medical career. Each one of us practitioners has different ways to grapple with the ER and its exigencies. I've been fortunate that, in conjunction with the writing, my style, the thing that has kept me relatively sane throughout my career, has been an ironic, Borscht Belt-inspired sense of humor.

I think I've incorporated much of that into my writing. This love of humor mixed in with a variety of literary and film references, has continued to this day to amuse me and from what I'm told, amuse my patients and colleagues as well. I'm thankful for that jibing, Jewish jocosity that has helped keep me sane throughout my career.

Here was where I discovered how to handle the stress of this work, which was to be my writing stories of the people who came in. And now, since we are in real-time in this book, I will take you into the Bellevue ER with me. In fact, I am going to take you into many of the ERs I ended up working in. Herewith, just one at Bellevue.

CHAPTER 8

SENOR BELLIANOVSKI

I hadn't been working at Bellevue very long before I became aware of the rhythmic flow of patients and staff around the various treatment rooms splayed throughout the cavernous Emergency Department.

Whether it was the Eye Room, the Minor Trauma Area, or the Asthma Alcove in the back, each place had its particular pattern that varied according to the time and day of the week. But while most of those locations' rhythm was chaotic, there was a place where the rhythm was most regular, that seemed in fact to set the pulse for everywhere else. This was the cramped Charting Area, in front of the Big Room.

The Big Room (so-called because it was the largest and most central of all the treatment areas comprising the old Bellevue Emergency Department) was the place where the sickest of the many patients who descended on Bellevue were seen and cared for. Its Charting Area was where, like clockwork, each day at 7:00 AM or PM, Morning and Evening Sign-Out Rounds would occur. Winter or summer, chaos or calm, at 7:00 on the dot, there'd be an assembling of personnel. The incoming medical team would stride through the doors, eager and ready to plunge in. The outgoing crew, bleary-eyed and often ready to plotz, would shuffle over to join them and exchange information regarding the care of, and plans for, the patients who remained in the ER at the change of shift.

While it hadn't taken long for me to accommodate to these hours, one day a few months into my tenure at Bellevue, this rhythm was broken. Arriving early for Morning Sign-Out Rounds, I'd just taken my seat, unwrapped my buttered bagel, and was about to pop open the lid on my coffee cup when I was approached by one of the paramedics.

"Dr. Weinberg, I know you just got here but there's a patient that I was hoping you'd see. We literally just dropped him off."

She paused and then, watching me rewrap my bagel and turn to face her more fully, she continued, "He's an elderly gentleman who we found wandering the streets of Flushing in the middle of the night. When we picked him up, he appeared very confused, seemed only to speak Russian, and clearly had no idea where his home was."

I followed her to this man's gurney in the Big Room and was instantly struck by his dignified facial features and sparkling blue eyes, set off as they were by a two-day stubble and a great shock of wild, thick white hair. He didn't look like he'd been living on the street and was dressed in a clean, if unfashionable, brown sports jacket, wide yellow cotton tie, and blue checked shirt. He also seemed very alert, immediately locking eyes with me and smiling as I approached him.

Despite this encouraging initial interaction, I quickly discovered that we couldn't communicate at all. I made several unsuccessful attempts to connect through words and gestures and was trying to decide on another approach when Annie, a young Irish nurse who'd also just arrived for the morning shift, approached me.

"Doctor, I know someone from the lab who speaks Russian. I just called her, and she is going to come talk with him. She only has a few minutes before she has to start her work up there, though."

When the translator appeared, I watched as she and my patient conversed in Russian. With her help, I was able to ask him a few brief questions and have him assent to my putting in an IV and drawing blood. Despite her assistance though, he was still unable to provide his name, date of birth, or address.

After she left, the Spanish-speaking EKG technician appeared and as she prepared him for his cardiogram, squeezing out the white, gooey electrode gel onto his chest, I started to banter with her en Espanol, as was our habit.

"Ah, que bueno que usted habla Espanol," my patient burst in. "How good that you speak Spanish!"

"Que increible que podemos hablar," I responded, thrilled and relieved that we suddenly had a way to communicate. "It's incredible we can speak to each other."

"Where are you from?" I asked.

"Argentina."

"No, I mean now. Where do you live?"

He had no response.

"How about your name?"

We tried this several times, but all I got was a garbled, unpronounceable, Eastern European-sounding moniker.

"Donde nacio? Where were you born?" I asked, sidetracked by the pleasure of being able to converse with him.

"Rusia."

With this, he began a ten-minute monologue on his early life, his training as a chemical engineer, and how he fled Russia in the 1930s. He told me his religion: Catholic; and politics: lapsed Communist. But as far as the present was concerned, it seemed as if it didn't exist.

I ordered a CT scan of the brain. Normal. His lab tests came back, also normal. By now, the Big Room was filling up, the morning's surge building, bringing its attending sounds and smells and heartbreak. Yet through it all, my patient sat calmly, observing everything, still unable to help provide me an answer to what had happened to him, his name, or if he'd left anyone behind.

Feeling that there was no more I could do and knowing he clearly needed to stay in the hospital for further evaluation, I spoke to the resident from the on-call Internal Medicine team and got him admitted. His diagnosis would be Altered Mental Status.

Realizing he'd soon be taken to a medical bed, possibly unattended to for hours by the busy team, I decided to make one more attempt at solving the puzzle of who he was and if perhaps there was someone I could notify.

"Como se llama?" I asked again.

"Me llamo Viktor."

"Y su appellido?" Your last name?

I'd asked it several times before. Now he produced the name: "Bellianovski."

Or at least that's what it sounded like.

I knew that behind the Big Room, on the way to the Walk-in Clinic, in the still quiet Social Services Office, there were some random phone books from each of the New York City boroughs stacked in a closet. I raced back there, found the one from Queens, went to the Bs, and rifled through its battered pages. Bellincoff. *Well, it is in Flushing*, I thought. (This was not the actual name.)

I ran to the phone. "Hello, this is Dr. Weinberg from Bellevue Hospital," I said to the woman who answered the call.

"Yes?" Her voice seemed to go up an octave.

"I have an elderly gentleman here..."

"My father, you have my father! He went out for a walk two days ago and never returned."

One-half hour later, Mr. Bellincoff's medical team came down. As I watched they wheeled him out of the Big Room into the busy corridor. And out of the corner of my eye, I saw a middle-aged woman walking briskly down the hall towards him. Bringing the entire procession to a halt, she leaned over the stretcher and gave her father a tear-filled embrace.

CHAPTER 9

FIRST, DO NO HARM

Being at Bellevue/NYU was a tremendous learning experience and after being there for four years, my father (who now ran the Radiology Department at Irvington General Hospital) in New Jersey told me that the administration there was looking for an Emergency Department Director.

I applied but didn't have a New Jersey license and because I was a foreign medical graduate, the State Medical Board was making it hard for me to obtain one. I arranged a meeting with the secretary of the Medical Board in Trenton, and my father came along for support. I will never forget sitting in Ms. Caroll, the board's secretary's office, and her questioning my official documents.

My father said he would vouch for them, and Carroll turned to him and asked, "Why should I believe YOU?"

She knew who my father was, at that point the president of the New Jersey Radiological Society among many other statewide affiliations, and I was flabbergasted, and embarrassed for him, at this incredibly disrespectful remark. Furious and thwarted, we left, and I wound up having to hire a lawyer to get my license. I ultimately met with the full

Medical Board and just before the job offer was going to be rescinded, I was granted the license to practice medicine in New Jersey.

I knew the town of Irvington well as it was close to South Orange, where I'd grown up. It had always been solidly working class but now had evolved from white, ethnic to largely Black, urban ghetto, indistinguishable from neighboring Newark.

Interestingly, during the 1940s, Irvington's white working-class population had supported an active, aggressive German American Bund. The members had developed a worrisome habit of inciting racist and anti-Semitic attacks in the nearby Black and Jewish communities. One day in the early 40s, the Bund members found themselves famously receiving retribution. They were assaulted, and their building was trashed by a group of rough Jews. The group included Swede Mason, inspiration for Swede Levov in Roth's novel *American Pastoral*, Abner "Longie" Zwillman, a major Mob racketeer, and Al Miller, a tough trucking magnate who later moved across the street from us in South Orange. Apparently, the Bund mishegoss was swiftly curtailed after this encounter.

While at Irvington General, I saw gunshot wounds, horrendously disabled chronic alcoholics and drug addicts, and an array of patients with the problems one would expect in an aging population with a fraying social net.

One day, I cared for an elderly man, accompanied by his wife, who came in with crushing chest pain. It was clear he was having a heart attack, and as I was taking his history, he went into ventricular fibrillation on the monitor in front of me, falling back lifeless on the bed. I quickly gave him a chest thump with my fist and to everyone's amazement, brought him back into a regular heart rhythm.

The next day, I went to see him in the CCU. Now stable, he was sitting comfortably in bed, reading the newspaper.

I asked how he was doing, and he said, "I'm feeling great. Thank you for all you did. But I must tell you that as I'm sitting here it feels like someone punched me in the chest."

It was also at IGH that I met Milton Block, an ironic, eighty-plus-year-old man, who was an avowedly and unabashedly Communist doctor. He and I became great friends, and I soon learned that he was a wealth of medical and historical information. Every time he'd pass through the ER, he'd come over and talk to me and the bemused nurses about one topic or another that was at the front of his mind.

Among his areas of interest were the findings of the 1965 Kerner Commission, put together by Congress amidst the civil rights upheaval tearing through the country at that time.

Milton was fond of quoting from their conclusion, "Our nation is moving toward two societies, one black, one white—separate and unequal."

He also liked to talk about Major General Smedley Butler (recently played by Robert DeNiro in the film "Amsterdam") who, in the 1930s prevented a Fascist coup against FDR, led by, among others, Prescott Bush (grandfather of W). Milton loved to recite a quote of Butler's: "I spent thirty-three years and four months in active military service and during that period I spent most of my time as a high-class muscle man for Big Business, for Wall Street and the bankers. In short, I was a racketeer, a gangster for capitalism."

While many of our colleagues had disdain for him and his outspoken politics and ongoing critique of the healthcare system, I found him to be a provocative and kind father figure. Milton and his wife came into the city to have dinner at our loft one lovely evening while I was working in Irvington.

A few years later, I learned that Milton's wife had died, and his son, also an MD, had gone to see how his father was doing. To his horror, he found Milton dead from a self-inflicted gunshot.

I soon had to leave IGH. The ER had been taken over by a cabal of Filipino and Middle Eastern MDs, who naively thought there was money to be made by running an ER servicing a largely Medicaid and self-pay population, and I was told I was out of a job. I now had to look for work again and answered an ad in the New York Times (an unusual, but as it turned out, fortuitous, place to job hunt). After a quick exchange of phone calls, I arranged to meet with the Director of the Emergency Department at Holy Name Hospital, in Teaneck, New Jersey.

We decided that he would come into Soho where we'd meet for dinner at Amsterdam's, a favorite local restaurant. Unbeknownst to me though, and in retrospect something I should have realized, I went to see him leaving Ona at the loft stewing about the timing of this meeting. She had just come home from the hospital, discharged after recuperating from the abruption that had almost taken her life and Georgia's, in childbirth. She had left Georgia, seven weeks premature, in the neonatal ICU at St. Vincents that day. Ona was furious that I would abandon her for a job interview when she'd just returned home without our daughter.

It was clearly one of the cracks that had begun to develop in our relationship, along with a horrible schism that developed in her own family during her pregnancy and that led, among other horrors, to her father's sudden death a few months after Georgia was born. The only consolation was that he'd come up once from Florida, seeing and holding his granddaughter, before he died.

Oblivious to Ona's anger, I came back from the dinner meeting that night very excited. The director was articulate, funny, and engaging, and it sounded like Holy Name was a reasonable environment. Plus, the job promised a salary that I felt at this point in my career was finally commensurate with what I deserved.

The misunderstanding with my wife was seemingly patched up, and I decided to take the job. I soon discovered from my father that a med school friend was working at Holy Name. He had been in Guadalajara with Marc and I and had transferred to Cuernavaca when we did. We'd endured a lot of lunacy together in Mexico, creating a bond, and I was excited to learn of his experiences at the hospital where I planned to begin working.

What I quickly found out was that he'd just been fired, and I was being given his job. He was understandably a bit wary of going into all of the details, but never-the-less didn't exactly try to dissuade me from coming on board at Holy Name either.

What I only learned later, after I had already been working there for several years, was that the ER director had created a scenario where he'd hire a new physician at an hourly salary the first year, and then, if all went well, have them enter a partnership track. At that point, they'd start to get an increasing percentage of the monthly profits. After four years, they'd theoretically become full partners.

Up till the time where I was hired, this had never occurred, however. This was because that same director was also keeping files on the MD's alleged infractions and when the time would come for full partnership, he'd pull out those files and say, "Whoops! How can I make you a full partner when you've had all of these major issues and complaints?"

This is what had just happened to my buddy.

This had been the modus operandi, that is, up till the time I was hired. What I learned years later from a friend, who'd been president of the hospital's medical staff at the time, was that soon after firing my friend, the Director had been told in no uncertain terms, that if he pulled that move again (it had occurred several times prior) that he would lose the contract, no longer be the Director.

As I said, I wasn't aware of this at the time, and did, though with some rocky fits and starts, become the first full partner, a job I kept for 22 years.

I also became aware, not long after this, that the Director had run another job ad in the New York Times. This one, though, attempted to draw New York docs to the more pristine, AIDS and drug-addict-free environs of suburban New Jersey. Lewis (Goldfrank) found out about the ad and read him the riot act. The ad quickly disappeared.

Holy Name was a tumultuous, increasingly busy (not AIDS or drug addict-free) suburban, Emergency Department. So busy that after my 15th year there, the hospital built out a vast new ER. It contained several mini-command centers run by a growing number of MDs, scribes, and PAs. They had been brought on board to handle the robust census of patients who were showing up from throughout Bergen County, New Jersey, and beyond.

The director turned out to be otherwise good, meticulous in record keeping, medical education, and navigating the hospital politics. I learned a tremendous amount from him and my colleagues.

And my relationships with many of my fellow doctors, the PAs, nurses, and later on, scribes gave me tremendous pleasure. I love teaching and as much as anything else, trying to show people I work with how to be as caring and humanistic as possible.

It was also where I started to fully realize the power I had, in those first few moments of a patient encounter, to turn a situation around, often with humor. To bring a frightened patient, afraid they are dying, out with a joke, lighten things up, puncture the tension and fear, and move things in a better, more healing, direction. Because I'd always felt that our minds had so much control over how bodily processes went down, I realized that I, as the one in charge, the Attending Physician, immediately radiating confidence and authority, and often, when I sensed it was right, humor, had the ability, especially in those first fraught minutes, to take things in a positive direction.

I also found out I didn't have a poker face. I'll never forget one patient, an elderly man in his 70s, who came in with chest pain. As I was talking to him and beginning to examine him, I looked at his cardiac monitor and saw he was throwing all kinds of dangerous heart rhythms.

"Am I going to be ok, doc?" he asked suddenly, intently examining my face.

I quickly looked back from the monitor.

"Why do you ask?" I replied.

"Because the look on your face just changed, and it made me very worried."

I had to laugh and then, immediately thereafter, also had to break open the code cart to quickly pull out and inject him with an anti-arhythmic drug that fortunately abated the abnormal tracings I was so intently watching on his monitor.

But probably most important of all that happened at Holy Name was the relationship I evolved with the nurses. I quickly came to realize that on many occasions, they were able to save my medical behind, alerting me in the middle of the myriad patient issues I was dealing with about something I missed and had not thought about regarding the many people who were in my care.

I realize now that because of my quirky Jewish humor and (sometimes too) laidback style, my relationships with the nurses, as well as the PAs and scribes, seemed to extend deeper than that of my colleagues. My use of Yiddish was also intriguing to them at this avowedly Catholic hospital. One day I went to a local sign maker in Soho and had them make a three-foot-long plaque with an expression I had come up with, using Hebrew letters that could just as easily be seen as English characters.

The sign said, "Don't hock the Doc," and it was my humorous way of admonishing the nurses not to hock or harass me when I was feeling overwhelmed. It hung by the nurses' station for many years until I was fired, and it now sits above the door in my guest bathroom in Old Chatham.

Interestingly, one of my most enduring friendships to this day is with Dr. John Poole, a (former) staunch Republican with whom I'd have frequent shouting matches or debates in the ER at Holy Name. They began in the Bush 1 era, through Clinton, Bush 2, and early Obama. Despite our seemingly diametrically opposing points of view, we developed a great respect for one another as MDs.

One day when Georgia was about 7 years old or so, she was visiting me in the ER, waiting for the shift to end for me to take her home. John walked in, saw her, and immediately, using air quotes, looked Georgia in the eye and said, "Conservative Republican". Georgia didn't respond, but as we walked out to the parking lot, she turned and said, "Dad, I have a question. If John Poole is a Republican, how come he wants to help people?" I immediately realized she understood an important concept of American politics.

A few years later, I had a patient in the ER during the Bush 2 era when John was the surgeon on call. The patient had a surgical issue that needed outpatient follow-up, and I sent him to John's office. The patient had no insurance, and when John's nurse asked him how he was going to pay, he told her (based on a prompt I'd given him when he was discharged from the ER), "Dr. Weinberg told me to let you know that George Bush will cover the bill."

The nurse was horrified until she relayed this message to John. Even now, this encounter still brings a huge smile to his face and mine.

The shifts at Holy Name were originally 7:00 p.m.-7:00 a.m. or 7:00 a.m.-7:00 p.m., though over the years more shifts were added to accommodate the ever-booming patient volume. Half the shifts we all had to do were overnight. I was reverse commuting from Soho in lower Manhattan during rush hour. Sitting in bumper-to-bumper traffic on the West Side Highway and over the George Washington Bridge to Bergen County, made those shifts especially difficult. In addition to my biorhythms being constantly messed with, when I worked nights, I'd have to leave two hours early to get to the hospital on time. Frequently, I'd arrive just before 7 PM and walk in to complete ER chaos. My food options had to be well-chosen to help get me through the night in a reasonably healthy manner. I'd also grab a nice iced latte on the way in and frequently replenish it throughout the waning hours of the shift with the not-quite-as-nice hospital coffee sitting out all night.

When the overnight shift ended, I'd find myself sitting in rush hour traffic going back into the city at 7:00 a.m. or so, desperately trying to stay awake. One technique I developed was listening to Howard Stern, whom I hated at the time, on the radio. My anger at his self-indulgent and sophomoric bullshit was usually more than enough to keep me going. Another was by imagining myself as the Humphrey Bogart character in They Drive By Night. I'd do as Bogie did on his long drives as a trucker up and down the California coast and keep my left arm hanging out the window, the bracing cold air on the arm enough to keep myself going. Fortunately, after several years, a room was found for us overnighters to sleep in in the morning after our shift ended. This allowed us to nap for at least a few hours and then wend our way home midday when there was no more traffic to deal with.

Other times, I'd ride my bike to the hospital, as I found that it didn't necessarily take much longer than the drive would, and I'd be pumped up by the time I arrived. Also, the rides along the bike path leading up to the George Washington Bridge were good for putting me into the headspace I needed to enter the 7:00 p.m. fray.

I was taking piano lessons at this time as well and often would leave home even earlier (neither Georgia nor Ona was often around) and use the grand piano in the quiet hospital auditorium to memorize a Bach cantata I was learning. It was meditative and was another way to put me into a balanced place when I entered the chaos at 7:00.

The bulk of my following ER stories were written during this time, some nearly fully written at the moment if I had time, or if not, the next day when things were still fresh in my mind. Many were in the form of quick notes jotted down of dialogue, beguiling or disturbing moments, intriguing phrases from patients (one man whom I suspect had a schizotypal personality disorder, came in saying he had a problem with his "budnocks" each time he went to "secrease").

I wound up spending twenty-two years at Holy Name. While there, I also worked at a few other ERs in NJ and Upstate New York, earning a bit more to pay for our loft, lifestyle, and Georgia's private school. It's also where I started doing house calls to that end as well. Often, I'd be notified about a patient needing to be seen as I was finishing up an ER shift. I'd get my supplies and head into the city, stethoscope, otoscope, penlight, and IV start kits at the ready, so I'd be prepared to evaluate and treat any of the foreign tourists who'd fallen ill on a trip to New York.

Herewith are the stories from Holy Name and those house calls.

CHAPTER 10

THE MAN WHO HUGGED ME

Late one busy Friday afternoon, the physician's assistant (PA) I was supervising approached me with a question about one of the patients she was seeing.

"Ken, please take a look at this guy and see if you think we should scan his head."

As we walked over to see him in the back of the emergency department (ED) (it was such a busy day that he was being examined in the room usually reserved for incoming cardiac arrests), she told me that he was there for a head laceration he'd sustained in a fall the day before. She was concerned because he said it had happened during the evening after he'd had a few drinks and now, at about 4:00 pm the following day, she thought she could still smell alcohol on his breath.

I appreciated her concern. Anyone who has spent any time working in medicine knows the potential land mines littering this patient's situation: alcoholic liver disease causing clotting problems, multiple falls after alcoholic blackouts, seizures, and hidden blood trapped inside various cavities in the skull and brain. Where in this landscape would our patient be?

Sitting on the gurney was a very pleasant, casually dressed man in his mid-40s. I introduced myself and examined the wound on the back of his head. It was about 2 inches long and deep enough to require staples to put it back together, but in the scheme of things didn't appear too serious. In addition, although I agreed that he still had a stale alcohol odor on his breath and seemed a bit out of focus, after speaking with him and doing an evaluation, I felt that he didn't need a CT scan of the head. What he clearly needed was to have someone talk to him about the real issue that had brought him to the ED.

As I found out, he was a man with a full-time job and a family; a very smart man with all the classic signs of substance abuse: denial, injury, self-destructive behavior, and defensiveness. How many times have I seen this in the ED? How many times have I tried to talk with someone? How many times have I not? We talked and I told him what I saw. I felt he was already clearly so deep into a behavior pattern which this time had only caused him a minor head injury, but was leading him toward much more serious, irreversible problems. The PA then came and stapled his head laceration, and I said goodbye to him as he headed out the door.

The following Friday morning, I was working, and at about 7:30 the triage nurse came over and asked if I would see a patient who'd come in to have his staples removed. I walked to his bedside and after a moment or two, prompted by his very warm greeting and handshake, I recognized my patient of the week before. With a huge smile on his face, he said,

"Hi, doc. I just had to shake your hand!"

As the nurse and I stood there, he continued, "I just want to tell you that what you said to me last week and the way you handled the situation really turned me around. You know when you think that maybe there's a problem, but you kind of put it aside and go on, you don't realize how it is? Well, after you talked to me last week, it hit me. I realized that I really did have an issue with drinking. I won't say that I stopped completely – on New Year's Eve, I had a beer, took out my telescope, and looked at Jupiter and that incredible full moon – but I really feel like a changed person. I am so grateful to you for taking the time to talk to me and for the way you pointed out the pattern of my behavior. You really helped me, and I think this issue is over for me."

As I took out the staples, we talked about our love of stargazing and about how the sky had been that New Year's night, and he got up to go. As the nurse looked on, he turned and embraced me in a heartfelt bear hug.

CHAPTER 11

WIND TUNNEL

Working the ER is an assault on the senses. The sound of an ill, frightened infant, screaming uncontrollably as she rolls in on the ambulance stretcher; the sight of a deep scalp wound, skull exposed stark white against the red and gray splotches of torn flesh; the feel of an abscess filled with pus and ready to burst, or the smell of hemorrhagic stool, passed by the alcoholic whose stomach ulcer is oozing blood, all waft and commingle as the work day unfolds. Fortunately, most of the time these sensory attacks percolate just below the surface, not affecting one's concentration and workflow, but sometimes, unexpectedly, they burst into consciousness, triggering such strong emotional responses that they bring things to a grinding halt.

After working fifteen years as a full-time emergency physician, I thought that I'd become inured to these visceral attacks, no matter how strong. I believed I'd seen, felt, or smelled it all.

One hectic winter afternoon, I was proven wrong. It started subtly at first, something nearly subliminal. Then a particularly foul and unfamiliar odor erupted, permeating the entire ER. It seemed to be emanating from a new arrival who'd just meandered past us. I had finished sewing a laceration and was walking back to my desk when this occurred.

"Ken, why don't you finish your charting on that patient's laceration?" suggested Margie, my physician's assistant. "I'll go find out what this is all about."

Margie had worked with me for several years. She was a little dynamo and before I could even turn around, she had run off, like a hound on the scent of a quarry, her nose leading her to a cubicle in the back of the ER.

Ten minutes later, she returned. The edges of her mouth were curled down, and the skin on her forehead was crinkled.

"I need your help on this one," Margie said, as she shook her head slowly back and forth.

"What's the scoop?" I asked, curiosity and repugnance swirling around in my brain.

"Patient's last name is Y. Her husband brought her here, and insisted that she come today. She has the most amazing tumor I've ever seen. After examining her I recommended that she be admitted. She agreed but freaked when I mentioned surgery and now, she's balking at even staying in the hospital."

As the attending physician in charge, it was now my turn to visit Mrs. Y. Walking back to her cubicle I recalled prior cases where a patient would clearly be ill to my clinical eye but would refuse to recognize the seriousness of the problem, sometimes angrily challenging my diagnosis and treatment recommendations. I thought of one man I'd seen recently who'd been experiencing several hours of chest pain at home. He'd finally been convinced by his wife to come to the hospital and when I saw him, he was pale, sweating profusely, clearly uncomfortable as he sat on his stretcher. I'd gotten an EKG, then told him gently but firmly that he was having a heart attack and that we needed to act right then to prevent any further damage to his heart. Before I finished my sentence, he'd pulled off the cardiac electrodes, jumped from the stretcher, and bolted out of the ER, running past me, the nurse, and his astonished wife. Five minutes later he'd been brought back in from the hospital parking lot in cardiac arrest.

I guessed, per Margie's observation and my own olfactory response, that Mrs. Y's condition had to have its own extreme, yet similar, sense of urgency, tinged with that same lack of acceptance. That she would contemplate leaving the ER without treatment for this seemed evidence of either dementia, psychosis, or deep denial.

I considered these possibilities and a strategy I could use to convince her to stay while I walked back to her room. As I entered the cubicle, I first saw Mr. Y, wringing his hands, pacing, eyebrows arched. By contrast, his wife was sitting calmly in a chair, harlequin reading glasses perched on the bridge of her nose, perusing a *Ladies Home Journal*.

Her voice was light, almost bouncy.

"Thank you so much for coming back here, doctor. Margie said you'd give me your opinion on how I should proceed."

"We need help bad, doc" interjected the husband. He stared directly into my face, eyes opened wide in frustration.

I looked again at Mrs. Y. She was an elderly woman, missing most of her teeth, yet stylishly dressed and speaking with what struck me as aristocratic assurance. Her contradictions were as evident as her medical condition. She sat, exuding an air of faded elegance, as well as a skunk-like fragrance I'd never encountered. It arose from a tumor on the right side of her head as large as the head itself.

"Mrs. Y," I began, trying as best as I could to hide my incredulity, "how long have you had this growth on your scalp?"

"Oh, about a year or two, I think," she responded sweetly.

I tried to imagine how she and her husband had been able to tolerate this unbelievable invader of their space for any period. It was a tremendous mass, well covered by skin and patches of hair, its weight causing her head to list a bit to starboard. Despite having left her scalp largely intact, the tumor was oozing a yellowish, viscous liquid from the several rents it had obviously caused in the dermis as it grew beyond even that pliable tissue's ability to expand. I looked from Mrs. Y. back to her husband. He appeared to be in his late seventies, with attire and a demeanor that conveyed a sense of command. He was wearing a hound's tooth jacket and rep tie, had on a Rolex watch, and manicured nails. I marveled at his apparent tolerance of his wife's persistence in not dealing with this.

I thought again of the man having the heart attack and a few other extreme cases of denial I'd experienced before. But those cases at least had some nuanced subtlety, enabling me to understand how the patient and family could have refused to acknowledge the problem. I could see no nuancing the severity of Mrs. Y.'s issue. I clearly had to convince her of the need for immediate and aggressive treatment.

Breathing through my mouth as a shield from the smell I continued my conversation, trying to mix authority with compassion.

"I understand how difficult this is for you, the problems and fear the growth of this tumor must have caused," I said. "The good thing is that surgery will take care of it."

I paused. But it really does have to be taken care of today."

"Thank you," said the husband. "It has been awful for both of us."

He took a deep breath (I knew not how) and exhaled slowly.

"Doctor," Mrs. Y. said, "I'm so afraid of the surgery. Won't it be very painful?"

"No. They'll put you to sleep and when you wake up it'll be gone, done with." I paused once more. "You've been extremely lucky that this thing hasn't burst, or given you blood poisoning." I hoped that stressing this would be the ultimate motivator, forcing her to make the decision to no longer live with this alien co-occupier of her head.

She sat silently for several moments, and I watched as her gaze seemed to turn inward with concern and anxiety and then outward to me in reluctant resolve. Forcing a smile, she finally spoke. "Okay. I know that you're right. Would you please notify my doctor? I want him to get me the best surgeon in the hospital if I'm going to go through with this."

I walked from her room to call John M., her primary care physician. On my way to the phone, I realized that I had just learned something new about the boundaries of denial.

"I have Mrs. Y in the ER," I said to John when he came on the line. "She's got a rather large tumor on the side of her head."

"Is her husband with her?" John asked.

"Absolutely. I doubt she'd be here if he hadn't persisted and brought her in," I replied. "Why do you ask?"

"Well, it's kind of ironic. The first time I ever took care of him," John answered, "he came into my office wearing a strange hat, very full at the top. The hat hid several tumors the size of golf balls on his head." John started chuckling and seemed to be waiting for my amused response.

"John," I parried back, "this one's much larger than a golf ball."

"My God," John responded, after a pause. "I always assumed she had a strange hairdo. Every time she'd come into the office with her husband, we all thought she looked as if she'd been in a wind tunnel and was covering her hair with a scarf."

Now it was my turn to pause. I felt like I could hear the requisite *bdrum bum bum* of the drumbeat after a vaudeville punch line.

"There was no wind tunnel, John. I can assure you of that," I answered. "She said she wants you to recommend the best surgeon in the hospital for her."

Three days later, I walked upstairs from the ER and went to visit Mrs. Y, who was now recovering from the surgery she'd had not long after I'd last seen her. In the operating room that day they'd successfully removed a benign, twenty-pound tumor from her scalp. She was making an excellent recovery.

As I peered into the room, I found her sitting in bed, watching TV. Bandages covered all of her head except the face.

"Dr. Weinberg," she said smiling, as she noticed me in the doorway. "Please come in." She extended her hand and brought me next to her. "I have to thank you for your firmness and the way you spoke to me the other day. I don't think I would have gone ahead with this if not for you."

"I'm happy your husband was able to get you to come in. He deserves a lot of credit as well," I responded.

"Oh, no. He actually wasn't the one who convinced me." She paused. "You know, that day was our fiftieth anniversary. We were in a Hertz office, getting a car to drive Upstate to celebrate. The man behind the counter forced me to come in. Refused to rent us a car." She paused and laughed. "Can you believe that?"

At that moment, the image of her, scarf strategically placed, pus and stench exuding from her scalp, maneuvering her way into a rental car and heading off up The Taconic State Parkway with her husband at the wheel, burst into my brain. I thought about the "wind tunnel," the depth of her, and her doctor's denial, and her husband's own tumors and realized what a debt of gratitude we all owed to the agent at Hertz Rent-a-Car.

CHAPTER 12

The Winds of Spring

One hectic Friday afternoon in early spring, I approached the stretcher of my next patient and noticed he had already been hooked up to the cardiac monitor. In a busy ER like ours, that was a sign that when the nurse had brought him in from triage, she'd had some concerns about his status, though not enough to have immediately interrupted me and taken me over to see him.

Glancing at the heart machine, I could see that his pulse rate was a normal 70 beats per minute. I looked at the patient as the monitor beeped regularly in the background and did a rapid evaluation just to see how he appeared. While he was obese and had a depressed, listless look on his face, he seemed to be resting comfortably on the stretcher. My impression was that he didn't seem ill, nor could I tell why he had been put on the monitor. As I looked at the triage notes, I saw that he was fifty-five years old and from his name, his features, and his accent, I guessed he was from the Middle East. The notes also showed that his blood pressure had been slightly low when he came in (though it had normalized when I saw him), and he had a low-grade fever.

As we spoke, he told me the reason he had shown up that day: "I've been feeling a bit weak for the last day, not a lot of energy. My appetite is okay, but I just can't seem to get moving. Feel a bit dizzy."

As I examined him, I was struck more by his flat, sorrowful affect than by anything on his physical examination. "Weak and dizzy" is one of the ER practitioner's most hated phrases. It can be heard from any patient with an impending stroke, sepsis, dangerously low sodium or potassium, to the hysterical, anxious somaticizer.

My patient now seemed fine, but there was that initial low blood pressure and low-grade fever I had to consider. I checked his blood pressure again and found it to be 80/65, low, especially for a 200-plus-pound man. I felt like he probably had a viral illness and some dehydration, so I decided to put in an IV, draw some routine blood tests, and watch him for the next few hours.

While walking to my desk to write the orders on him, I noticed that Alan Felsen, that day's on-call physician, was sitting in the ER talking to one of the nurses. Efficiency and timing are so important in keeping the flow in the ER as smooth as possible, so I walked over and discussed this patient with Alan. I knew he would want to know about the patient sooner rather than later to make his own workflow efficient as well.

After our conversation, Alan obligingly went to see the patient as I sat writing orders. He came back and said he had decided to admit the patient for observation.

The rest of the afternoon took on its typical frantic crescendo pace and knowing that Alan was caring for this patient now, by the time I left at 7 PM, my "weak and dizzy" patient had been lost to me in the rush of later events.

I was off for the weekend, and Ona, Georgia, and I drove straight up to Ithaca to stay with my brother Neil and his family when I left work.

The next morning, I was sitting on the deck of Neil's home in the woods, drinking my coffee and casually reading the New York Times. I happened to notice a small item tucked in the back in The Metro Section. It talked about two patients who had been admitted late Friday to the teaching hospital located near the one I work at. Their diagnosis was botulism!

I knew immediately it was my patient. But who was the other one? Botulism? What had I missed? Were they still alive?

As soon as I could, I called Alan. I was desperate to know how they had made the diagnosis and what had subsequently transpired.

And I was upset with myself for missing it. I did not, however, expect to hear what Alan had to say.

It turned out that my patient's blood pressure never came up in the Emergency Room despite multiple interventions and it became clear that the patient needed an ICU bed. Our hospital's critical care beds were all filled so Alan transferred the patient (and his wife who had come in later with the same symptoms) to the teaching hospital where he also had admitting privileges.

Early the next Saturday morning, Alan was making rounds in the ICU with his medical resident. As they discussed this particular case, the resident, a Coptic Christian from Egypt, realized that this patient was an Egyptian Copt as well. He immediately told Alan about a ritual that was widespread in Egypt and had been brought to the United States by the Coptic community here. It was known as Sham el-Nessim. Loosely translated as "The Winds of Spring," this was a practice that was celebrated at the time of Passover and Easter and historically predated those two festivals. It called for the burial of fish that were wrapped in paper in the earth. After two weeks, the fish were unearthed and eaten. In the age of Saran Wrap, however, the fish now were sealed in that airtight wrapping, creating the perfect environment for the growth of Clostridium botulinum. This is a bacterium that only develops when contained in a space that has no oxygen and that causes botulism.

As the resident described further details to Alan, he learned that every Springtime in Cairo, hundreds of people became very ill or died of this practice. Alan now realized that the practice had "surfaced" in the United States and through a serendipitous and fortuitous set of circumstances, had landed these two patients in his care. Because of the semi-indolent course of their illness, Alan was able to begin treatment quickly enough to save both of their lives, and through his subsequent extensive research educated me on this once ancient and ongoing disturbing practice.

Three years later, once again in springtime, I was on duty in the ER. As I approached the bedside of my next patient, I recognized this same man. Despite his nearly fatal earlier episode, he had apparently continued his religious practice. And now he had come in once more, with the same ingestion, same time of year, and same symptoms! I was flabbergasted and couldn't believe that despite his prior event he'd apparently not understood what happened or was such a fervent believer that his faith overruled the potential risk to his life. I kept my mouth shut and began the treatment I now knew he needed. We quickly admitted him to our ICU so we could bring him back from the brink one more time.

CHAPTER 13

On Succos Reciting the Bruchas

"You have your yarmulke with you?"

"No," I said.

"Here then. Take mine."

I had to smile as I realized that it had been many years since I had had any yarmulke with me. My smile lingered, and I recalled a day when I'd reached for my wallet in the pocket of an old brown sports jacket and instead pulled out a personalized, gold skull cap from the bar mitzvah of my nephew Ben, then a twenty-eight-year-old adult. Both jacket and skullcap were long since gone.

My smile turned into a chuckle as I watched my interlocutor—a small, heavyset man with glasses, a beard, and a disarming demeanor - reach up, remove his own yarmulke and place the warm, worn, head covering on the top of my scalp.

It was the second night of *Succos*, the Jewish Festival of the Harvest, and I was in Crown Heights to do a medical house call on his nephew, a fourteen-year-old boy, visiting from Brazil, who had a fever and an earache.

I had been doing these calls for eight years, traversing the five boroughs of New York, and schlepping to the suburbs, on subways, bicycle, foot, and car, seeing tourists in hotels, hostels, or the homes of relatives. Once, I had to meet a patient with a sore throat inside a busy Starbucks on 23rd and Third in Manhattan. Faced between the choice of evaluating her amidst a sea of caramel macchiatos or in my car, I opted for the latter. We walked out to my Volvo station wagon and went inside. I leaned over the gearshift between the seats, took out my penlight, and conducted the examination there.

These calls were a refreshing change from the work I had done for thirty years as an ER doctor, slower paced, and more under my control and the patients (who have called their insurance company which then contacts me) were always appreciative. Plus, it gave me a chance to see them, often in the context of where they live, fleshing out an important piece of who they are and making the experience that much richer for us both.

As the uncle and I spoke that day, we had just entered the *succah*, or arbor, a small open room off the back of his kitchen (he had decided, after walking into the house and seeing me with his nephew, that I needed to say the Succos prayers). His succah was fashioned (in a rather ersatz way) with random tree branches and exotic fruits and vegetables to look like the setting the ancient Hebrews had used to celebrate the harvest thousands of years ago.

"Now what will I use for a yarmulke?" the uncle wondered out loud.

I turned and joined him in searching the arbor frantically. As we explored the tiny, makeshift setting, I was struck by its disarray. Succos is one of the most joyful holidays in the Jewish calendar, but I didn't dare imagine what had taken place the night before. Chairs, tables, plastic soda bottles, dirty drinking cups, and packages of white bread were scattered amidst the branches, fruits, and vegetables.

I didn't see anything the now bareheaded uncle might employ, but he was vastly more resourceful than I was. In a trice, something in the debris caught his eye. Sweeping his hand to the ground, he plucked out a small black plastic bag, handles cut into its top. Picking it up, he put it over the back of his head, its handgrips sticking out from his ears.

While I marveled at his choice, it didn't surprise me when it wasn't a snug fit and he had to hold it in place so it wouldn't fall off. As he clutched the crinkling bag with his right hand, he grabbed the lulav and esrog in his left.

"Do you remember the *bruchot*, the blessings?" he asked as he handed me the gnarled plants. "Oh, and you need something to drink as well."

On one of the bare metal rental tables was a 16 oz. bottle of warm, flat Diet Sprite. "Josephine, can you get me a cup, please?" he asked of the large, older Black woman who had been watching these proceedings as she mopped the floor in the kitchen. She graciously complied, the Sprite was poured, and we were ready to proceed.

"Now, repeat after me," he began. "*Baruch, atah, adonai, elehainu melach ha'olom...*"

I had driven out to Crown Heights half an hour before this interaction took place. It was a bright October afternoon, and the early Fall air was still warm as Josephine let me into a modest brick row house with a white, plastic boxed-in sign over the door announcing its affiliation with Chabad, the Lubavitcher Hasidic movement.

My patient, redheaded and slight, had appeared, climbing the stairs from the basement where he was staying. He began speaking to me in Yiddish.

I responded in English.

He tried again, this time in Portuguese.

I answered in Spanish, and he smiled in acknowledgment.

Our mode of communication now established, we began to tackle the problem at hand ("earache") as we walked into the large, mostly bare, living room and settled onto a long, musty couch.

As I took out my otoscope to examine his ears, I glanced around the room. There was fancy glassed-in shelving on one wall, filled with rows of books with gold Hebrew lettering. The rest of the space was bare and unkempt: a few old, plastic chairs scattered about, a battered credenza on the far wall, children's toys on the floor. Two young adolescent women reading from small, paperback prayer books hovered in the background. One appeared to be deaf. They were doing their best to ignore what was happening with their cousin.

Soon his aunt joined us. She was a short woman with a warm smile, a modest, gray dress, and a blonde wig.

"So? What does he have? What's wrong with my little boychik here?"

His aunt was concerned about him and was intrigued by me: A nice Jewish doctor who did house calls.

"Looks like a bad infection and sinus congestion," I said, pulling the black tip of the otoscope from his tender left ear.

"He needs antibiotics? They're expensive?"

"Nah. I'll write for generic."

"So, how much is that?"

"I'll bet less than twenty bucks."

"Do me a favor. Call the druggist. Find out for sure."

I picked up my Blackberry and punched in the number she gave me. "Is this the pharmacist? Yeah, Dr. Weinberg. How much for Bactrim DS #14?"

I waited a few moments. "It's $18. Is that okay?" I asked her.

"Boy, I hope you take Medicaid. I know a lot of people who would love to have you make house calls," the aunt replied.

As she spoke, I recalled my own experience sleeping in the basement of a different Lubavitcher household nearly forty years earlier. Having become interested in Buddhism and mysticism in my second year of college, I decided to return to my roots and explore Jewish occult practices. I phoned Herbert Weiner, the rabbi who had Bar Mitzvahed me seven years earlier. (And had officiated at my first wedding, a few years later, at the age of twenty-three).

Weiner had recently written a book, *The Wild Goats of Ein Gedi*, about his own burgeoning explorations in Jewish mysticism. After our initial phone call, I had gone to see him when I was home from college.

That day in his study Weiner told me about "encounters with Chabad". These were weekend introductions to the life of studying Kabbala (the mystical Jewish book) run by the sect headed by Menachem Schneerson. Schneerson was the legendary Hasidic rebbe who believed in Baal teshuva, the concept of bringing secular Jews into the Orthodox faith.

I had signed up and taken the subway out to Crown Heights on a Friday afternoon that winter, slept in a basement with ten other long-haired Jewish heretics like myself, and then on Saturday morning walked alongside the rabbi I was staying with and his family to the gender-segregated shul for Shabbos services. I subsequently learned that while most Hasidic men are rabbis, few are rebbes. Only learned men with a following are deserving of that title.

When the prayers in shul were finished, the men adjourned to a room adjoining the chapel and sat at a long table packed with and pressed in by, the faithful. They passed around schnapps and listened raptly as Schneerson intoned in Yiddish about that day's Haftorah and worldly events. As the schnapps went round, and round, and glasses were filled, and downed, we partook of the tradition of raising our cup and toasting, giving a L'chaim, "To Life," to the Learned One, whose followers believed him to be next to God. The other non-Hasids and I were told that if you caught the rebbe's eye, it meant good luck for you.

As I watched one of my fellow apostates repeatedly grab the bottle and begin to lose control, I raised my own cup and caught a wink from the great man. I never learned any of the secrets of Kabbala from my hosts, left early, and disappointed later that day. My luck never really turned bad, however, and the experience has stayed with me. Now, here I was once more, back among the Hasids.

In the intervening years, I had actually developed a certain antipathy towards them and the other Orthodox Jews I frequently had to treat in the ER. They seemed arrogant and ruled by magical thinking, and I felt their disdain toward others, especially non-observant Jews like myself. I had come to feel that they always wanted fellow Jews to bend the rules for them: I would get calls on Friday afternoon from Orthodox Jewish doctors telling me about their patients coming into the Emergency Room. They'd call, not to tell me anything in particular about the patient, but instead to ask me to see them before other patients so they could get home before Sabbath sundown.

But this rabbi and his family seemed different. After reciting the *brucha*, shaking the lulav and esrog, drinking the Diet Sprite, and returning the rabbi's skullcap, we ambled back into the house and it was decided that the family had to take my picture with them, then ply me with Lubavitcher literature and finally give me a coin collection box with a picture of Rebbe Schneerson on it even though he had died many years before. They told me that every year on Succos, tens of thousands of Jews come from all over the world to Crown Heights, celebrating for two days, drinking and dancing in the streets till morning, and begged me to join them that night.

Unfortunately, I had to leave. Had another house call to do in Midtown and I was worried about the traffic. But as I walked out the door with Josephine (who smiled at me like a co-conspirator,) I found myself surrounded by hundreds of Hasidic men, women, and children, walking in streets brightly covered in fallen leaves. The energy was palpable as they strode from their stores to their homes and synagogues. As I drove off, I felt I had completed a cycle and sensed that something had unexpectedly changed inside of me when I went to examine my fourteen-year-old Brazilian patient in Crown Heights that day.

CHAPTER 14

TOXIC TURKEY DAY

It's five o'clock on Thanksgiving morning. I've been working since 7:00 p.m. the night before, and even though it's been a pretty uneventful night in the ER, I just want my 12 hours to be over. I can barely wait for my family to come in from Soho, pick me up in my Northern New Jersey hospital, and allow me to drop off to sleep in the backseat of our Volvo station wagon as we drive two hours upstate to start a nice Thanksgiving Day weekend in the country.

As I sit reading the early edition of *The New York Times* online, I hear two patients register at the front desk. From the garrulous voice of one of them, a woman in her early twenties, I sense that she was there for something that occurred sometime earlier in the night, presumably after she'd been drinking. The other patient, a man in his late forties, had come in because he woke up and began to painlessly urinate blood after a urological procedure he had done the day before. To help pass a kidney stone he had a stent placed in his right ureter, the tube carrying urine from the kidney to the bladder. He called the doctor, Dr. F., who did the procedure because he hadn't been told that it was fairly routine to pee some blood after manipulation of the urinary tract. Now Dr. F. had instructed him to come to the ER.

Told him and the wife that he'd meet them there. I get up to evaluate the young woman, and knowing Dr. F. and his ways, I ask the nurses to call him about his alleged plan to come to the ER at 5:00 a.m. Having been through this scenario too many times in the past I want to confirm if this is the case or if he wants me to see his patient instead.

Sure enough, as I stand speaking to the other patient, Abby (who, it turned out, had fallen and hit her head as she struggled with her boyfriend over a bottle of beer), I overhear the nurse speaking with Dr. F, the urologist.

"Okay, doctor, yes, we'll admit Mr. G and I'll have the ER doctor see him. Yes, I understand you aren't planning on coming in until later on today."

"Would you let the patient know about that little deviation, please?" I say to the nurse as I peer out of the curtain of Abby's room.

Fortunately, Abby only has a minor cut on her head needing some ointment and a tetanus shot, and has someone who will drive her home and watch her until she sobers up. I tell her and Susan, her sister, my assessment and plan, reassure them that nothing serious has happened to her brain, and attempt to leave to see the patient peeing blood.

"Oh, by the way," Abby says as I begin to leave the room, "I don't think I can go on with this."

I look at her and Susan.

“That’s all right, forget I said that,” she adds, having witnessed the glance I shot at her sister.

Susan looks at me and shrugs, “She doesn’t mean anything by that. She’s just a bit drunk. She’s said that before and when she sobers up, she always denies that she’s feeling that way.”

“Okay. And you will watch her, Susan?” I ask.

“Yeah, she’s lived with us for two years,” Susan smiles. “We’ll all be together for the next several days.”

“Well, I can’t believe that doctor!” Mr. G’s wife says through gritted teeth as soon as I walk into their room.

“He seemed so concerned, called us back, and told us to meet him here. Now he only wants to get blood drawn and won’t be here until later on today.”

“How are you feeling?” I ask, trying to move the conversation forward, afraid of what I’ll say about Dr. F and his behavior. “Any fever or chills?”

“No, I feel fine. I wouldn’t even have come in if he’d talked to me after the procedure and told me that I could expect this to happen.” He pauses, then, “I should have known there was a problem when Dr. M referred us to him. While we were sitting in F’s waiting room, he was having a loud argument in front of several of us with the wife of a patient, saying something like ‘I work very hard. Don’t you make any accusations like that to me!’”

I look at the patient’s chart. He’s otherwise healthy, has no fever, and takes no medicine other than the antibiotic he'd just been prescribed after this procedure, done to help him pass an unwieldy kidney stone. I examine him and give him the requisite punch to the kidneys to elicit the pain associated with a kidney infection and he doesn't flinch. In fact, he looks very good to me, not toxic, as we would say of someone brewing a nasty infection after a procedure, certainly not someone who needs to be admitted on Thanksgiving Day.

"Is Dr. M around?" I ask. "I can call him and see if he can help us here."

"Give him a call please," says G's wife. "I think he also should know about this because this is the guy he uses for referrals."

Twenty minutes later, as the man's blood tests come back, Dr. M calls. My patient first speaks with the doctor and then I get on the line.

"So that's the situation," I say. "He looks fine, his white blood count is barely out of whack, he's already on antibiotics and now he's going to need to be admitted, to stay here on Thanksgiving Day."

Dr. M hesitates. "Okay, that doesn't seem fair," he finally says.

"I'll call Dr. F myself and see if we can get him to do something."

By now it's 7:00 a.m. I go to evaluate Abby one last time so she could be discharged. As I walk into her room, she motions for her sister to leave.

"Doctor," she says, her speech still slurred from the eight beers she'd imbibed earlier, "I'm very depressed. I meant it earlier when I said I might want to hurt myself."

We discuss this situation again for several minutes. "Do you have a therapist? Are you thinking about hurting yourself now?"

"No, I think I'll be okay, but my therapist died two years ago, and I don't know how to find someone who's good I can continue therapy with."

"I'll give you the name of our psychiatrist. He's very good, very nice. You can see him on Friday. In the meantime, go home today, you need to sleep. You've been up all night. See how you feel later. You can always come back if you're feeling that way when you sober up."

I walk out of the room once more and see Susan, the sister, again. I discuss this with her as well and she concurs.

I change into my street clothes from my ER scrubs. I'm aching for a few relaxing days up in the country. But first, I walk by my patient with blood in the urine.

"Doctor thank you so much for intervening. I know how politically difficult this can be," says his wife. "And by the way, what is your specialty? Where is your practice?"

"You're in my practice right now. I'm trained as an emergency physician," I say and pause before adding, "but I've been forced to become a human relations specialist as well."

CHAPTER 15

Sunday's Sorrow

It all began as a straightforward sign-out.

"Bed Two is Mr. Barbuto. He's 35 years old; has a history of gallstones," I was told by my partner Brian. "Looks like he's jaundiced. His doctor saw him in an Urge-Care center this morning for right-sided abdominal pain. Then his pain went away so they sent him home."

"And he's in our Emergency Room now because...?" I asked, glancing into the cubicle and smiling at Mr. Barbuto. It was 7 o'clock Sunday night, and I had just begun working the 12-hour overnight shift, learning about all the patients I'd be responsible for and where in the various stages of their workups they were.

"Well, the pain returned so his doc told him to come in to be seen by us," Brian said as we walked towards Bed Three. "We're waiting for the results of his blood tests to decide what to do."

With that summary we continued our rounds, moving on to the remaining cubicles to discuss the other patients. Brian and I finished up and he headed home. Just as I was on my way to see my first new patient, Marianne, the nurse taking care of Mr. Barbuto, approached me.

"Bed Two's blood tests are back," she said, handing me three white sheets of paper from the lab. "None of the numbers look critical but there is some sign of inflammation of the liver."

I turned and called Herb Schwarz, Mr. Barbuto's physician.

"I have Mr. Barbuto here. Your partner saw him this morning…" I began.

"Yeah, that guy's been to our urgi-center several times in the last few weeks. Each time he shows up with vague *mishugee*. Absolute nonsense! What's going on now?" Herb asked, the rough tone of his voice conveying annoyance.

"He's got belly pain again. Plus, his liver enzymes and white count are a bit high. I think he needs to be admitted."

"Fine, we'll admit him but keep him down in the ER. I'll be there in an hour. Oh, and order a CAT scan of his abdomen," Herb added. "I don't know what the hell is going on here."

I hung up with Herb and went to see Mr. Barbuto. I wanted to discuss his blood tests and tell him our plan, including the prep he'd need for the scan.

As I walked into the cubicle, I got my first real look at him. He sat on his bed, a slender man in his mid-forties, white, with short, dark brown hair. A grey hospital gown covered the top of his blue jeans. When I approached the bedside, he looked at me and managed a thin smile.

Two women were with him. One was an attractive Hispanic woman with thick black hair pulled back into a tight ponytail. She sat in a chair to the right side of the bed, feet up on a stool reading a local newspaper. An older woman, whom I later learned to be his mother, stood by the other side of the bed. She had tinted glasses and upswept gray hair and was gesturing with her arms as she spoke in a thick Italian accent, her voice barely audible. When I entered the cubicle she turned towards me, raised her arms to her chest and stopped talking.

"Your tests aren't too bad," I began, "looks like there is some inflammation of the liver or gallbladder, though. I just spoke to Dr. Schwarz, and he wants us to admit you and get a CAT scan of your abdomen tonight. It'll take about three hours between the prep and scan itself and then we should have a much better idea of what's happening."

"What else can I do, doc?" Mr. Barbuto asked. "This has been going on too long, and I need to get to the bottom of it."

I noted his tone of resignation, nodded to the three of them, and needing to catch up on the new patients, headed back to the nurses' station.

"Would you mix the contrast so we can scan Mr. Barbuto's belly?" I asked Marianne.

"Why's Schwarz ordering a CAT scan?" Marianne asked, looking straight at me, "We can get an ultrasound of his gallbladder in a half hour and have an answer."

I'd wondered the same thing.

Marianne shrugged her shoulders. As I looked back at her I thought about how she and I had been through this kind of thing before and how we shared an acute sense of irony regarding the roles we sometimes played in the ER. We knew how and when to advocate for the patient if we disagreed with their attending physician, and when to back off and say nothing. We had spent many long, trying, and tumultuous ER nights together over the years and I valued her clinical judgment, her sensitivity, and her opinion.

Doctor Schwarz arrived forty-five minutes later. He was a heavyset man, with a full, round belly and a scowl on his face. He went right into Mr. Barbuto's cubicle and almost right away I heard muffled voices arguing from behind the curtains.

After about ten minutes Schwarz strode out of the cubicle. His face was red and as soon as he saw me, he stomped over to where I was standing.

"Ken, Barbuto's a pain in my ass. His wife and mother have been hocking me for weeks about this belly thing. I ordered the CAT scan just to get them off my back, plus, you never know..."

Frowning in frustration, he marched to the desk and wrote his admitting orders.

I stood for a moment thinking about what I'd just witnessed and felt sympathy for the Barbutos. As I turned to walk away, I noticed Mr. Barbuto's mother looking at me from behind the curtain.

"Doctore!" she called in a harsh whisper, motioning for me to come into the room and close the curtains.

"Doctore," she repeated, sotto voce, once I was inside. "We no like this doctor."

"Yeah," her son added, "I saw him a few weeks ago. I was having the same pain, and he didn't do a damn thing for me."

"Dr. Schwarz said he might have hepatitis, but they never followed up on it at all," said his wife.

She grimaced.

"Today we saw his partner, and he did an ultrasound. It never even got read. It feels like neither of them knows what's going on with my husband. Or even cares."

She paused and then added, "Isn't there any way you can help us, maybe find us another doctor?"

"Boy, I don't know," I replied, taken aback by this request. "You already have a doctor. He's here right now. This makes me very uncomfortable." I hoped that my firm tone would convey my unease.

"Well, we feel very uncomfortable with him. We didn't realize it would be Dr. Schwarz coming in," his wife responded, a scowl wrinkling her forehead and pulling back the corners of her mouth. "Can't you help us?

Unsure of how to deal with this I said, "Let's wait and see what the CAT scan shows. As soon as I get the reading I'll come back, and we can try to figure something out."

“Thanks, doc, we really appreciate that,” Mr. Barbuto said.

He extended his arm and gave me a firm handshake. I walked out of the cubicle hoping that the scan results would clear things up and we could make a decision that would put them more at ease.

With that I began to put the Barbutos in the back of my mind and continued seeing the new patients who'd arrived. The night was so busy, and I had other. personal issues revolving around in my brain, otherwise I think I would have anticipated what came next.

Three hours later, Marianne gestured towards me.

“Mr. Barbuto's scan has been read. I'm just pulling the interpretation up on the computer here.”

We brought over two chairs, sat, and perused the description displayed on the screen. It was mostly bland nonspecific radiological terminology: areas of low attenuation, inflammatory changes, streaking in the large intestine...

Then came the last line, no longer bland but bleak. As stark and specific as it could be: “Multiple 9-centimeter mets to the liver.”

Metastatic cancer! I felt my heart drop. I felt like Schwarz, and the vague history I'd gotten about the last few weeks, had led me astray. I felt like the impact on me at that moment would have been less if the Barbutos had experienced a more caring attitude from Schwarz (and I wondered if Schwarz hadn't suspected this result when he'd ordered the scan). And I felt that because I'd been put into the role of the Barbutos advocate here, I'd just been devastated myself.

Yet, how was I going to give them this horrible information? Despite the last few hours I'd spent with the Barbutos as their doctor in the E.R. we barely had a relationship, and my own personal problems, not far from the surface on this night, made me feel less centered than I usually would be when delivering difficult news. I also knew that many patients would want to receive news like this only from their primary doctor. It felt like walking into the Barbutos cubicle with this information would be akin to a punch in the face to them; if I knew them better there would be so many more paths open between us that could help ease the shock I was sure this would cause. But here it was 2 in the morning, and I'd told them I'd come back with the results...

"What are you going to do?" Marianne asked, pulling me out of this reverie. Her blue eyes had narrowed.

"God, I don't know!" I paused for a second. "I can't remember the last time something hit me like this."

I took a deep breath.

"Why the hell did I say I was going to give them the reading instead of just getting him admitted?"

I stood and walked with Marianne to Bed Two. As we entered the cubicle and I looked at the Barbutos' hopeful faces, I wished my professional mask was fitting me better, wished I'd told them that they could just change doctors in the morning, wished for anything other than what I had to do at that moment.

"The scan is bad," I began, struggling to find the right words, and trying to adopt an empathic tone as I felt their expectant stares. "It shows cancer that has spread to the liver."

The mother gasped, her jaw dropping as her right hand reached back to cover her now wide-open mouth. Her knees seemed to buckle as she clumsily sank into a chair next to her son. Mr. Barbuto crumpled against the back of the bed, his head dropping to his chest as his hands began reflexively grasping the sides of the gray hospital gown. His wife sat, momentarily stunned, and then rose uneasily from her chair and took Mr. Barbuto in her arms, tears starting to pour down her cheeks. Her whole body quivered as she silently sobbed.

"Doctor, what is going to happen to my life?" The patient seemed to be shouting this at me as his wife squeezed him.

"Mr. Barbuto, we don't know exactly what this all means," I said. I was barely acquainted with the rest of his medical history. I had that one line from the CAT scan. One ghastly line. A virtual death sentence and now I'd had to pronounce it. I tried to be as gentle and compassionate as I could.

"There have to be so many more tests to really figure this all out." I hesitated. "I'm deeply sorry to be delivering this news. I think that it's the last thing any of us expected."

I found myself thinking about Dr. Schwarz again but continued, "This is agonizing. It's one of the worst things about the ER. Sometimes we get this terrible information that feels like it's just coming out of the blue. We can't put it into perspective."

"Isn't there something we can do about Dr. Schwarz?" the mother said between sobs as she turned to face me.

I watched as more tears began to roll down her cheeks. I was unsure what to say.

"Yeah," Mr. Barbuto growled, moving forward on the bed and freeing himself from his wife's embrace. "That *bumbatz* saw me three weeks ago. Maybe something else could have been done if he had started the whole workup then and hadn't freaking blown me off like he did." His voice quivered in anger.

"Okay," I said. I was relieved for even this temporary reprieve.

"I don't think it's necessarily true that that would have changed things. What I do know is that in the morning, Schwarz will bring in an oncologist, that's a cancer doctor, and probably a GI doctor. You might decide to use them more and deal much less with Dr. Schwarz."

The mom stood and came close to me, speaking in a pleading tone, "Doctore. I have a doctor here, Dr. Lorelli. Could we use him?"

"Sure." I eagerly jumped on this information. "Lorelli's partner is on tonight. I'll call him now and let him know what's going on. Tomorrow you can call Schwarz and tell him you don't want to use him anymore."

"But not before you've spoken to Lorelli himself, Mrs. Barbuto," Marianne added.

I looked over at her.

"Make sure that it's OK with him," she continued. "You have to be certain that you have someone who is definitely going to be your doctor before you drop Schwarz."

I found myself turning back from Marianne to the family. I felt the overwhelming sadness and pain in their faces as I watched them trying to take everything in. I felt my own pain, my sadness at life, and death, and the role I sometimes am forced to play in them as an Emergency Physician. I felt how this tragedy of theirs had bound me to them at a time when I was feeling very vulnerable myself.

And then an impulse seized me. I moved forward and reaching my right arm out, grabbed Mr. Barbuto and squeezed him. With my left arm, I reached for his mother and hugged her, and we sobbed together in silence. I thought about how much this had rocked me; thought about how, despite all my medical training, my 20 years of working in the Emergency Room, forced by the daily deluge of death and suffering to feel like I could deliver bad news only by keeping my distance, that something could have come along and knocked me down like this and just torn away my defenses. I thought about what it was with this situation: the warmth of the family, my feeling of shock at the CAT scan results, a protective feeling I'd developed for them, that caused me to react this way to news I've delivered so many times before. And then I thought about how being a doctor meant not simply keeping your mind open but your heart as well, and I realized that in that moment of spontaneously sharing the sorrow and tears and hugs I had found another way of healing, not from a textbook but from a patient in need.

CHAPTER 16

FUCKING HEADACHE

Deep into a tumultuous Saturday night, two men from the local volunteer ambulance crew burst through the doors of our Emergency Department. They whizzed their stretcher through the background pandemonium, passed a barking, croupy three-year-old boy on Bed 5, neatly avoided the vomit from a 40-year-old alcoholic woman on Bed 3, and screeched to a halt at the side of the last empty bed, number 6. As they began unbuckling the straps securing their patient to the stretcher, they told me about the man they'd just brought in. Offhandedly, the older of the two crew members (wearing a green John Deere cap) tossed out a brief report to me: "Yeah doc, this guy called us complaining of a headache. Sounds like he did a little bit too much drinking tonight."

"By the way," his younger partner allowed, "it seems like he doesn't speak our language."

"What language does he speak?" I asked.

"I think he speaks Korean if that's any help," the younger one replied as he and his partner turned to go.

“Any family with him, or anyone who can translate?” I shouted through the din at their now retreating figures. “How about his vital signs?”

“Nah, no one came with him,” John Deere shouted back and then apologetically he added, “Look, we’ve gotta go, got another call to get to!”

On that note, he and his partner quickened their pace and with the squawks of their walkie-talkies and the clicking of their stretcher wheels fading off down the hall, they were gone.

Apart from the nurse’s aide now quickly taking his vital signs, my new patient sat unattended on Bed 6 for the better part of the next hour while I ran over to Bed 8 to suture a nasty scalp wound an eighteen-year-old kid had incurred in a street fight, and then went off to the Quiet Room. In that location, generally used to isolate and evaluate psychiatric patients, I found a delusional, agitated, thirty-nine-year-old homeless man who’d been brought in by the police because they’d found him walking down the street kicking over every garbage can he came in contact with on his travels through town.

Finally, I got around to my patient on Bed 6. I walked into his cubicle, its lights dimmed by the aide because of his headache, and got a good look at him for the first time. He was a middle-aged Asian man, dressed casually in a brown crew-neck sweater and jeans, with a thick shock of straight, short, gray-flecked black hair. While he seemed to be comfortable as he sat on the gurney, eyes open, arms folded across his chest, I was struck by what seemed to be the contortion of his round face. Its features appeared all tightened up and I immediately wondered if this was from the discomfort of the headache that had allegedly brought him in.

"Hi, I'm Doctor Weinberg," I said. "Sorry it took so long to get to see you."

He stared at the curtain I'd pulled closed when I entered the room.

"Can you tell me your name?" I asked, not sure if he understood me. Same blank stare.

Having seen many Koreans in the ER during my years there I thought I would use the one phrase I had learned and asked his name in that language.

"Kim," he said and then began a long, incomprehensible monologue in Korean to me.

Now it was my turn to stare blankly at him. "Can you tell me what happened to you tonight?" I asked, shifting back to my native tongue. No response.

I moved closer to his bedside and looked more attentively at him. I thought about what the ambulance crew had said and tried to sense if he had the typical wasted appearance and flat affect of someone who spent the night drinking.

"Can you close your eyes?" He did. "Now, can you open your eyes and follow my fingers?" He reopened his eyes but continued to stare at the curtain. "Could you try to squeeze my fingers?" I said as I put my hands by his, my index fingers extended for him. No response. "Can you tell me why you're here?"

Nothing. "What's bothering you?" I finally blurted out.

"Fucking headache. Fucking headache."

This disconcerted me a bit and all I could think to ask next was, "Have you been drinking?"

"Fucking headache. Fucking headache."

The words were said in a deep, angry monotone, clearly enunciated, but with a Korean accent so heavy that it made them nearly unintelligible.

Oy, now what? I thought, feeling stymied and uneasy. I looked over at his chart, sitting on the bedside table where I'd placed it when I came into the room. I glanced at his name, saw it actually was Kim, and then scanned down to the vital signs obtained earlier by the aide. No high blood pressure, no fever, I noted. No stiff neck, I felt as I tried to examine him as best as I could, taking his head in my hands and gently moving it backward and forward. Unlikely he has meningitis or a bleed in his brain. No bruises or swelling on his face or head. No signs of trauma anywhere. No alcohol smell, no smell of anything strange he might have ingested, I thought, getting up close to him, discreetly sniffing and anxiously scrutinizing my own brain as I tried to find any clue that could help me decide what was causing Mr. Kim's headache.

What do I do? He clearly needs a CAT scan. Should I call in the radiologist from home now and do it as an emergency? Or maybe, since I can't find anything really critical going on, I can give him pain medications, and if he feels better scan him first thing in the morning when the weekend radiologist comes in.

This was at a time in the mid-1990s, when, in the typical community hospital, to get a CAT scan in the middle of the night meant waking the on-call radiologist and having him or her come in to supervise the shooting and interpretation of the scan. There was a delicate process involved: knowing when to push this for someone who really needed an emergent scan and when to hold off, for medical and political, reasons. In that case, we'd wait till 7:00 or so in the morning when the daytime radiologist would normally come in, and make sure they'd do the scan first thing as they arrived for their shift.

Here it was, four o'clock on a Sunday morning and I was stuck. I'd been a full-time ER doctor for about ten years, used to working on my own, trusting my clinical judgment, making decisions, and moving on to the next case. I wanted to do what was best for this man, but the language barrier made me feel like I was dealing with a black box. I thought about how critical words were in getting a flavor of someone's illness; was grateful for my fluency in the Spanish and French languages, but at that moment, I wished that I knew so many more.

My unease worsened as I began ruminating about how unnerving Headache Patients could be. Fearing an unwanted headache about to descend on me, I decided to get another opinion.

"Lissa," I called to his nurse. "Mr. Kim in Bed 6 seems to have a pretty bad headache but I can't find anything wrong when I examine him. He understands so little English and my Korean being what it is, I can't really get a good sense of how serious this is."

Lissa walked to the bedside. She had grown up riding on the ambulance crew and had worked in the ER for several years. I respected her judgment.

"How about giving him some pain meds," she asked as she examined him, "and seeing how he responds? You can always wake the radiologist up to come in and scan him if he doesn't get better."

"That's funny. I was thinking the same thing," I concurred, smiling.

I wrote an order for Toradol, a non-narcotic IV pain medication. Lissa administered it, and he seemed to feel much better.

Within minutes, he stopped repeating what I'd come to think of as his mantra, his face seemed to loosen up and he fell asleep. Feeling better myself now, I went off to see the new patients who'd arrived and just before 7:00 a.m., called the tech and radiologist to make sure they scanned Mr. Kim as soon as they arrived at the hospital. Before I left the ER, I told the physician coming in to work the day shift my concerns about this case and went home feeling

I'd done the right thing, and Mr. Kim would be taken care of appropriately.

Twenty-four hours later, I came in to do the Monday day shift and before I even had a chance to take the lid off my coffee cup, Charlie S., one of the staff radiologists, called me.

"Kenny, I'm reviewing the CAT scans from yesterday," Charlie said in a panicked voice. "There was a patient who had a scan first thing Sunday morning that was read as normal. It was not a normal study!"

The CAT scan he was talking about was Mr. Kim's. It turned out that the part-time weekend radiologist had missed something critical on the images, images that showed abnormal blood in his brain, a subarachnoid hemorrhage.

"Subarachnoid. We missed a fucking subarachnoid!" I slid into a panic myself. The words reverberated in my own brain as the nurses and I raced to find Mr. Kim's chart to see what had happened to him on Sunday and more importantly, to see if there was a way we could locate him immediately. We knew we had a time bomb on our hands, knew that two-thirds of all patients don't survive a bleed like this, and knew that he required emergency neurosurgery to save his life. As we searched, I kept thinking about how missing a "subarachnoid" was an ER doctor's worst nightmare.

We quickly found the chart, saw that Mr. Kim apparently had been feeling fine when he came back from his scan and had been sent home with our standard "Headache Precautions" Discharge Sheet (in English, of course.) As Charlie now showed me on the scan he brought over, Mr. Kim did not have a standard headache at all but instead, had burst an aneurysm in his head and literally bled into his brain, the elusive cause up till now of his expletive headache.

Surveying this chart again, all of its data appearing in such a different light to me now than when I'd last seen it early Sunday morning, I found to my surprise that the ambulance crew had actually left a phone number for Mr. Kim. I dialed the number in a frenzy, my heart racing, not knowing if anyone would answer, not knowing if they'd speak English, not knowing if Mr. Kim was even alive.

A woman answered and I explained how serious the situation was, and how Mr. Kim needed to come back to the ER right away. I hung up the phone hoping that she understood what I was saying. We called for a Korean translator, and I then began a wait that was one of the longest and most agonizing half hours of my life.

Thirty minutes later, the doors to the ER opened and once more, let in Mr. Kim, now with his family of three.

"Dr. Weinberg?" Mr. Kim asked, smiling, as the group approached me. I nodded. "You called and spoke to my wife a little while ago, said something serious was going on with me?" All of this spoken in English that contained only the barest hint of an accent.

Trying to hide my shock I yelled to the charge nurse: "Eileen, Mr. Kim is back. Notify the OR and please call the doc who's on for Neurosurgery. Tell them it's urgent!"

I guided Mr. Kim and his family to the now-empty Quiet Room so we could prepare him for surgery. "Mr. Kim, I'm so happy to see you, so happy you seem to be okay, so happy to be able to really talk with you," the words and feelings seemed to burst out of my mouth all at once as we walked into the room.

As he put on the hospital gown I handed him, Mr. Kim turned and informed his family in Korean what I'd just told him. We all sat down together as the nurse came in to chart his vital signs and draw his blood.

"Mr. Kim," I said, "when you came in Saturday night with your headache, a very serious event occurred. A blood vessel burst and leaked blood into your brain. From the way you seem now, the bleeding has at least temporarily stopped but it could bleed again at any minute, and you need to have surgery as quickly as possible to prevent that from happening."

Mr. Kim seemed incredibly poised and dignified as he listened to me, as we prepped him for the OR, for the daunting, prolonged surgery from which he would have a complete recovery. I sat next to him and thought back to Saturday night, to the ambulance crew, to my frustrations at my inability to penetrate the "black box." I thought about the complexity of the brain's language center, and how the tidal quality of the ebb and flow of blood through it had caused the damage I'd seen evidence of on Saturday night. Now, because of the incredible resiliency of Mr. Kim's brain, the language center's function had been at least temporarily restored, giving him a lexicon of much more than the two words of our language I last heard him use. I also thought about the black box of my own language and cultural barriers and how they had so nearly cost this man his life.

CHAPTER 17

Is Healthcare a Human Right?

Not long after I started working at Holy Name Hospital, in the early 1990s, I attended an Emergency Medicine conference in Chicago, hosted by ACEP, the American College of Emergency Medicine. ACEP is the mainstream, original organization created to advocate for ER doctors and had been organized, not too many years before, as Emergency Medicine was just being recognized as a legitimate specialty. The organization held several well-attended conferences throughout the year, and I always looked forward to them.

The conferences are fun, and very informative, with a plethora of well-stocked booths and many top-notch speakers. They are always a chance to meet and schmooze with colleagues and spend time in a different city. This conference had so far been all of that, but, in addition, in between lectures, it inadvertently led to a chance meeting between me and my old girlfriend from medical school, Helene.

This was the first time I'd seen her in 15 years, since the nightmarish weekend when she'd broken my heart. She'd ostensibly come to NYC then to attend my brother Neil's wedding party, but once she landed at LaGuardia and I went to pick her up, it was obvious that our intense medical school romance was wrenchingly over. The relationship had begun in Guadalajara and continued through the crazy and frustrating time when we transferred med schools to one in Cuernavaca and deepened after several trips to Oaxaca and the beach at San Blas. It had persisted through our move to Park Slope in Brooklyn, where we'd rented an apartment and been immersed for months studying for Part 1 of the National Medical Boards.

Helene had then been able to transfer back into the third year of medical school in Wisconsin, and I'd stayed in New York, but we kept in close touch. I thought we were both still in love, and this was to be our first time seeing each other since she'd moved to Madison.

The day before the wedding, she'd flown into LaGuardia and as we sat in the car in the parking lot, it became clear she'd moved on. We cried and hugged for many long minutes after she blurted out that she'd fallen for another man. Painfully, she got out of the car, took her luggage, went back into the terminal, and caught the next plane back to Madison.

Our surprise meeting, now in Chicago, was bittersweet, though ultimately healing.

As I learned, after med school, Helene, too, had become an ER doc, and she was now the Director of an Emergency Medicine department in that city. After an awkward several initial minutes (not helped by the fact that one of my ER partners from Holy Name walked over to us in the middle of it), she invited me for lunch, took me to her office in the hospital where she worked, and we more or less got past the pain that had occurred so many years before.

After Helene dropped me back off at the convention hall, and still reeling a bit from our chance encounter, I continued my tour through the many booths set up at the conference. Included among the array were those selling the latest emergency medicine books, many others showcasing professional recruiting organizations and companies selling the latest innovative gadgets. These included things like medical Crazy Glue (actually developed during the Vietnam War to instantly, though temporarily, glue back together the body parts of soldiers mangled in the field); patented devices with gadgets that pushed deep up, and expanded into, nostrils to stop nosebleeds; or others that plucked foreign bodies out of ears.

Amidst the booths, I chanced upon one for a group called Physicians for a National Health Program. PNHP had been formed recently, and it advocated for Single Payer, or government-run health insurance. The group proposed a plan for folding the entire U.S. population, cradle to grave, into the Medicare program, i.e. Medicare for All.

The organization had been started by Doctors Steffie Woolhandler, David Himmelstein, Oli Fein, nuclear physicist Len Rodberg, and others, including nurses and social workers, at a Quaker retreat in New Hampshire in 1986. The group was working on policies first proposed by Teddy Roosevelt, later elaborated on by the Communist (at the time) influenced American Public Health Association, blocked in Congress in the '30s by the racist Southern Democrats, proposed again by Harry Truman (and Michigan congressman John Dingell) in the '40s and '50s; and blocked by the AMA throughout all this time well into the 60s, with the passage of Medicare. Len Rodberg had worked on a single-payer plan with Congressman Ron Dellums in the '70s and finally, after the group put together their proposal in '86, they published an article in January of 1989 in *The New England Journal of Medicine* outlining the details. The supportive editor of NEJM at the time was Dr. Arnold S. Relman, who wanted to take things one step further and institute a National Health Service, with all MDs being government employees).

Another early member was Dr. Quentin Young, Martin Luther King's Chicago doctor. Young had opened the national PNHP office in Chicago, and the members I met that day were part of that cabal. Of interest is that Young's partner, Dr. David Scheiner, was, for many years, Barack Obama's doctor. In fact, Obama had said, during the major political maneuvering that went on as he finally pushed through Obamacare, that if he had his choice for how to handle the vast bureaucratic mess that is our healthcare system, it would have been single-payer, Medicare For All.

At the booth that day in Chicago, I was struck by the fact that these docs were thoughtful, left-wing, fellow travelers, and I spent the rest of the afternoon with them (mercifully leaving my Helene experience behind). I began getting educated about the nuances of health insurance far beyond what I knew before and immediately joined the organization.

As soon as I got back to New York, I became involved with the New York Metro Chapter in Manhattan.

The rationale behind what PNHP was and is proposing is that Medicare has a 3% overhead compared to the 30% overhead of private insurers. It's efficient and has no one looking to siphon off funds to pay exorbitant executive salaries or any concerns about showing profits to shareholders, as private insurance companies do. Along with the universal coverage mandate, it would allow patients access to any medical practitioner and provide drug benefits to all while using the tremendous leverage and bargaining power of the United States population to negotiate drug prices with Big Pharma. With all of that in mind, it felt like a no-brainer. A striking additional point in its favor was the fact that the United States is the only industrialized country in the world that doesn't have some form of single payer.

At this point in my career, I had seen enough of what was going on every day in the ER, and how that reflected what was happening outside the hospital as well: people delaying care for fear of the costs; my colleagues asking me when I'd want to admit a sick patient to them, if the patient had insurance; or those same colleagues being unwilling to see a patient in follow up in their offices because of the type of insurance, or lack thereof, that the patient had. It had long been clear to me that things needed to change, and single payer seemed like the smartest way to bring that change about.

As soon as I became involved with the New York group, I found that they had lively, provocative, and informative monthly forums, at which I became a regular attendee. After a couple of years and some pointed remarks I made at some of those forums, citing my own perspective and experience as an ER doctor, I was asked by Joanne Landy, who was the executive director at the time, to be on the board. I was honored and immediately accepted the position, which I still hold, though in an honorary status.

The people who participated in these forums comprised a very diverse group of MDs, nurses, educators, financial consultants, and other healthcare professionals. (One of the members was Lewis Goldfrank, who spoke at one of our forums and later was honored at the yearly fundraiser Gala. PNHP felt he deserved recognition for all he'd done to provide quality health care for everyone who came through the doors at Bellevue.) In addition, PHNP's annual conferences, held at locations across the country, were always well attended and included among other things, workshops on policy, social action, and public education, with speakers such as then *New England Journal of Medicine* editor, Marcia Angell (a PNHP supporter also, and published documenter of the mendacity of Big Pharma).

When Obama later became U.S. President and he, and then Congress, were debating how to reform the health insurance system, experts of many persuasions were asked to come to the White House to proffer their opinions. Disturbingly, no one advocating for Single Payer was invited. Immediately, word went out to our members, and doctors in white coats began protesting in front of the White House, demanding the single-payer option be included in the discussions. These optics were not what the administration wanted, and they quickly went on the offensive. Late in the afternoon when the White House discussions (and protests) were taking place, Dr. Fein (who'd started the NYC chapter after the first gathering in New Hampshire) got a frantic phone call from Obama's people. They asked if he could please hop on the next Metroliner down to D.C. and add his voice to the conversation.

That got the docs parading in front of 1600 Pennsylvania Avenue to disperse and stop the embarrassment their presence was causing Obama. While Oli did hop the train, meet Obama, take his time advocating for a single-payer system, and give regards to Obama from Quentin Young, it turned out that his schlepping down there was nothing more than a face-saving gesture for the President and his advisors.

The debate then moved to Congress. Katie Robbins, one of our fearless members, attended the hearings run by then-Senator Max Baucus from Montana. In the middle of the goings-on, she stood up and said, "Senator, I'd like to talk about Single Payer."

Baucus was outraged at her effrontery, immediately called over a Capitol police officer, and had her arrested, thus squelching any further mention of Medicare for All in the Capitol.

While Oli was able to quickly intervene to get her released from the Congressional hoosegow, unfortunately, nothing more occurred to move the needle or debate in favor of single payer at that critical juncture.

In my nearly thirty years of involvement in PNHP, I've learned a tremendous amount about our dysfunctional healthcare system, been trained in civil disobedience (in a workshop given at the office of The War Resistors League on 4th Avenue in downtown Manhattan), lectured around New York State about Single Payer to med schools and to the New Jersey State legislature. I've had many debates with right-wingers, outraged at the concept of "Socialized Medicine," and soon learned that the best way to stop the accusations they made was for me to ask, "I have a question for you. Do you think health care is a human right?"

That oftentimes will stop them as it's hard for a physician to say that she or he wants to deny medical care to anyone. Other arguments they make are that the lines are long in Canada or England. It's a debatable point, and I often will say that lines are long to see specialists in this country as well; those two countries spend 9% of their GDP on healthcare, whereas we spend 17%, and they have better outcomes. Starting with Margaret Thatcher and then subsequent British administrations, they have done all they can to gut and cut funding for the largely beloved National Health System. Choice of provider is frequently cited as something that "socialized" systems make difficult, but anyone who has had to change health insurance and loses their PCP knows how common an event that is here. Another critique is that making the drug companies less profitable by forcing them to negotiate drug prices with the federal government (as Biden did recently) takes away their incentive and funds to do research. That is another canard, as Dr Angell documented in her book, *The Truth About the Drug Companies*. When they say a large percentage of their costs are R&D related, in truth, the largest percentage of their profits has traditionally gone to wining and dining physicians. Much of the research done in this country is at federally funded medical schools. As I mentioned, Medicare is vastly more efficient than private insurance companies, with their large bureaucracies of coders and deniers of care, plus the need to show profits to shareholders and pay large salaries to the CEOs. With the profits of Big Pharma and private health insurers, they can lobby hard for the status quo. Much harder than an organization like PNHP, nurses, or teachers' organizations who also are single-payer advocates.

My first time out on the single payer lecture circuit, speaking at an afternoon conference on health care in Monticello (Upstate in The Catskills), I appeared on the program with Congressman Maurice Hinchey. Hinchey was a progressive Hudson Valley legislator and very supportive of single payer. I felt honored to be on the same platform as him and to get to meet and talk to him when we finished. (His daughter is now our state senator, has worked with me on medical cannabis outreach, and supports her father's stance on single payer.)

After Congressman Hinchey and I spoke, a line of attendees came up to engage in further conversation with us. One of them, a tall, middle-aged man who'd been waiting patiently, finally approached me and said, "You know, watching you speak just now, the way you talk and the gestures you make, remind me very much of the doctor I see when I'm wintering in Sarasota, Florida."

It took me a moment to understand and then I asked, "Oh, you mean my brother, Marc?"

In fact, he did. I had never considered it before, but I immediately understood that my two brothers and I had grown up exhibiting many of the same gestures and mannerisms, and it felt very touching to realize it.

In 2006, I attended an evening lecture on current political events at Barnes and Noble in Union Square. I attended because one of the speakers was Paul Krugman. At that time, he'd been advocating for Single Payer in his *New York Times* columns, and he spoke on this topic that night. When the lecture ended, and Paul had finally peeled off from the last of the hangers-on, I trailed him down the escalator and out into the street. I stopped him and asked if he'd be willing to give a talk to PNHP. He seemed amenable and told me to contact his secretary.

Sure enough, not long thereafter, we arranged for him to speak at a PNHP meeting on National Health Care. The response to the announcement of his talk was so overwhelming that, instead of the smaller space we used for our monthly forums at the Beth Israel complex on Union Square, PNHP had to book The Church of the Incarnation on 35th and Madison to hold the crowd. It probably wound up numbering about 500.

I excitedly attended with two fellow travelers, my cousin, Norman Shaffer, and Sara W. (Dr. Rita Charon from Narrative Medicine was there as well. She commented to me later that she felt that the atmosphere was too Left/labor, which she thought had detracted from PHNP's attempt to move the needle on National Healthcare.) Nevertheless, it was a great event. Krugman gave a rousing speech and Oli had me stand in front of the assembled masses to acknowledge my making it happen. As we left the church I felt as if I'd really played some role in trying to advance the cause.

Later, through my involvement with PNHP and because we had a spacious Soho loft to accommodate them, we held two major fundraisers there. One featured Bruce Vladek, who'd been head of CMS (Centers for Medicare Services), and the other brought in Congressman John Conyers, the sponsor of a long-standing bill to create Single Payer National Healthcare. (As soon as Conyers came into our space that day, he asked me to make sure we had Miles Davis playing in the background. It was a request I was happy and able to accommodate.)

Over thirty years of involvement in PNHP, I've met tremendously dedicated people and been challenged by my colleagues about the workings of our healthcare system and how to improve it. Among other interventions, I subscribe to the concept that if national healthcare were to be implemented, it should be run in regions like the five regions that run the Federal Reserve, though in the opposite of the Reserve's pyramidal, top-down, manner.

Because of the horrific, nearly universal fear those of us in healthcare have about lawsuits (something that would inevitably come up in discussion of national healthcare) with the help of Len Rodberg and Joanne Landy, I wrote a comprehensive piece about how we should be instituting no-fault malpractice insurance, as several other industrialized countries do. This could thereby change the dynamic between MD and patient, removing the fear my colleagues and I have about lawsuits in any of our encounters with patients.

Hopefully, I've opened up minds over the years, about how critical having health care coverage to everyone in the country is. This could allow people to stop worrying about being able to access health care when they need it.

After traveling to other countries with national health insurance I was struck by the fact that, in those countries, if a person gets sick, they immediately make an appointment to see their practitioner, and don't even consider putting it off. In the United States, on the other hand, if people get sick, they begin to think of ways to ignore it, not deal with it, hope it'll go away, or take matters into their own hands. I find myself constantly disturbed by those diametrically opposing situations and resultant attitudes.

I'll never forget a patient encounter I had that exemplified it in such a stark manner.

When I first started working in Urgent Care, I had a patient, an otherwise healthy thirty-year-old man, come in for treatment. I saw him on a Monday morning and immediately was struck by the multiple cuts and bruises he had on his forehead. I was surprised and asked what had happened to him.

"I was riding my bike Saturday night, went over the handlebars, and hit my head. I think I blacked out for a few minutes," he replied

"What did you do?" I asked, assuming he'd gone to the ER and had a CT scan. "Well, I don't have health insurance, so I went home and asked a friend to stay with me to make sure I was okay. Now I'd like some help in dealing with these cuts on my head."

When the Occupy Wall Street events were occurring, some of the MDs and nurses from PNHP went down there. We helped set up a medical tent and treated the protestors who were camping out. During this time, we organized a march up Broadway to Union Square (one of many we had) for Single Payer. There was a lot of press coverage, and I was interviewed, in my white coat, by a reporter. That night, the Keith Olbermann Show devoted its entire segment to the day's demonstration and the topic of national health care. I was notified by several friends (one of whom fortunately taped it) that my interview, angry yet measured, led off the segment.

Another very meaningful march we were involved with was on May Day around 2004. Some of the *hibakusha*, elderly survivors of the bombing of Hiroshima and Nagasaki, had flown in to take part in the antiwar protests. They would be parading up 6th Avenue to Central Park for the demonstration and they'd reached out to PNHP when they got into town. Many of them were now frail and elderly, some in wheelchairs and they were looking for practitioners who'd accompany them on the march. I went with board members

Dr. Dick Pearson and medic Jay Kallio; Dick and I in our white coats, Jay in their medic uniform. When we were introduced to the group, they all applauded us. I was embarrassed by this, turned and bowed and thanked them for coming, for all they had gone through. Georgia and her friend Clara joined us on the march, and I have a wonderful picture of the two of them walking up 6th Avenue, next to one of the smiling Japanese survivors. The man is holding a signature crane in his hand.

Through the many years I was involved with PNHP (living Upstate almost full time now has precluded my ongoing ability to be significantly involved), I've come in contact with incredibly dedicated people: a nurse now 100, who'd cared for the sick in China in the 1930s; people willing to put their bodies on the line for this cause; Assemblyman Richard Gottfried who'd been trying for years to get single-payer instituted in the state (and who interestingly years later I enticed to sit on a panel we held at the Friars Club to talk about Medical Cannabis, something he'd also been pushing, finally successfully, for about 20 years at the time); Dr. Mary Bassett, a member who was honored by PNHP, not long before she became the head of NYC Department of Health, prior to being appointed NY State Health Commissioner by Governor Hochul; marched next to Reverend Al Sharpton down Broadway to City Hall; maybe even brought some of my colleagues over to our side.

When I keep on asking my skeptical conservative colleagues, "Is healthcare a human right?" I suspect in their heart of hearts that they do believe it is. I mean, isn't that what one gleans from the Hippocratic oath? As I write, though, this is still an uphill battle and the stakes have only gotten higher, though the opposition has questionably weakened, as it's clear that Obamacare has improved the lives of so many people.

I believe this shows that the government can, and should,. ensure that no one has that fear of a catastrophic medical expense, that one day none of my colleagues in the ER will face the frustration, outrage, and pain we see when people without health coverage show up ravaged by their inability to get the care all of us are entitled to. And we won't have to worry that when we speak to that surgeon on call to admit our patient with say, a bowel obstruction, the first thing we're asked is, "Does the patient have insurance?"

In writing this, I had long conversations with Drs. Len Rodberg and Martha Livingston, both long-time PNHP members, and forceful, articulate voices for pushing Medicare for All forward. As Martha and I spoke, I recalled a conversation we'd had many years ago, when I was voicing my frustration with the lack of progress we seemed to have made in making this happen.

Martha said to me then, "Kenny, we all need to recognize that we've got to be in this for the long haul if we're ever going to get it across the finish line!"

Thinking of that frustration I realized, after I ended my conversation with her, that one of the most rewarding things that I have gotten, in my thirty-plus years of being involved with PNHP, has been the ability to get to know and work alongside this group of smart, dedicated, humanistic people. Just being in it with them has been a reward in itself.

CHAPTER 18

JOSÉ DOE

Sometime in the early 2000s, the population of alarmingly intoxicated alcoholics who were transported to the ER where I worked seemed to grow at a rapid rate. The increase was largely made up of Hispanic men, and it coincided with an influx, in that period, of immigrants from Central American countries. There were disturbing parallels with so many of the other, earlier eras of large immigrant inflows into the country, the attempts at rational debate, and the dives into demagoguery that surround us now, once again, as I write this during the depths of Trump's latest provocations. (This was written initially during Trump 1.0. As I reviewed it during 2.0, I am horrified by how much he has, in his cruel, inhumane way, upped the ante.)

These men would be brought in by police or EMTs late on a Friday or Saturday night, after hours of voracious, bibulous indulgence. I'd find them when I came in to work at 7 the next morning, in a far corner of the Emergency Department, sleeping it off. This corner became an area of the ER most of us tried to avoid on weekends as we dashed from room to room because it seemed to always carry an odor of fetid feet, stale alcohol breath, and soiled, urine-soaked work clothes.

On these overnights, our medium-sized, suburban New Jersey hospital's Emergency Room would frequently have multiple beds lined up to accommodate these men in their various stages of intoxication. Most were from Mexico; most had no ID, and they all were apparently illegal immigrants. I had no idea how many actually resided in our area but learned that they all had come to the United States looking for full-time work. Yet, apart from the odd jobs they seemed to occasionally land would instead, at this point in their desperate lives, mostly wind up getting frighteningly drunk and be discovered in that state, in the street, or in other less likely locales. Because of their clearly stuporous, potentially dangerous, condition, they'd get picked up by the authorities and dropped off in the Emergency Department for our evaluation and temporary safekeeping.

This situation had evolved from the way things had been for countless decades where drunks would be brought to the local jails to sober up. The number of people brought to the "Drunk Tanks" who'd not been drunk at all, or who had serious medical and psychiatric issues that played themselves out with disastrous effect, had finally caused legislative and policy changes, very wisely, so that anyone with an altered mental state, even if they were stinking of alcohol would immediately get a medical evaluation. It was a humane and legally proper thing to do but the strain It put on Emergency Departments resources could be enormous.

Typically, these mén (I never saw a woman) would invariably spend the night, sometimes belligerent and shackled, or more often, just plain stupefied, out cold on their backs.

All of us who worked in the ER got to know them, did what we could when they came in, and then watched, helplessly, as they returned over a period of months or years, dying the slow, or sometimes violently fast, desperate deaths of those who'd lost their hope to alcohol.

Most came in anonymously as John, or José, Doe, barely able to stand let alone speak their names. They'd get varying degrees of medical scrutiny and most of the time, uneventfully sober up and leave sometime the next day. By then they'd have their legitimate names, Armando Raymundo, or Jesus Sanchez, finally placed on their chart. They told us, when they were sober, that most of them would depart from the ER and go back out to try to get jobs as day laborers.

It was understood that they'd stand in lines at designated street corners in the surrounding towns, waiting to be picked up by the American bosses who'd drive up and offer them work. The labor was either in construction or landscaping or doing other menial tasks that apparently our local citizens had no interest in doing.

Some actually seemed to occasionally save some of the money they'd make so they could send it back home. By the time they began appearing in the Emergency Room though, most had already been sucked into a cycle of earning, then spending, their hard-earned dollars on a late-night drunken spree, only to start it all again the next morning.

I would watch this, as an ER doctor, as the son of second and third-generation immigrants, and as a citizen watching the immigration debate unfold in the press and among the tirades of politicians. Just as today, the talking points were well staked out, both sides hardened, causing conversations that rarely seemed to address the human side of the situation: the desperate, dreary, daily existence of decent men who'd risked all to come to a place of greater opportunity only to find themselves exploited, abused and thwarted in their attempts to get a better life for them and their families.

Over a period of several years, as I watched the number of intoxicated illegal immigrants being brought to our ER climb, I also watched the neglect society showed them as they'd hide or sneak into the cracks and crannies of our country, littering the streets and empty lots in their stupors.

And I watched and intervened as I could when they came into my ER. One very hectic, early winter evening, one of these men, probably in his early thirties, was brought in by a busy ambulance crew. They were so busy that they only had time to tell us that he had been found, deeply intoxicated, at a construction site. With that pronouncement, they turned and sped out, on their way to another call.

This patient was so inebriated that he was unable to speak, and (as we later discovered) numb to any pain, as he was helped onto a stretcher.

He was initially examined by a Physician Assistant who found nothing of note, no obvious cause for alarm, just another Friday Night José Doe. But soon thereafter the nurse went back and checked his blood pressure, and found it was on the low side. Thinking he was dehydrated we placed an intravenous line and began giving him fluids. When, after a substantial volume of saline solution had gone in and the pressure hadn't risen at all, I went with the PA to his bedside and did a more thorough examination. The man was barely rousable from his stupor and yet still in no apparent distress as we poked and prodded, looking for reasons that his blood pressure was not responding. We quickly placed a second IV line, ran in more fluids and drew blood, ordered X-rays, and finally, a CT scan of his chest and abdomen.

It was through this scan that we discovered he had multiple broken ribs, a punctured lung, and a ruptured spleen. His stupor had clearly made him numb to his injuries and unable to tell us anything that might have caused them.

I hurriedly contacted the surgeon on call, and we made arrangements for him to be sent up to the operating room. As he waited to be whisked off to the O.R., multiple IV lines running fluid and blood to replace his own red cells oozing out inside him, his pressure slowly inching up, the ambulance crew reappeared.

Along with them came the police team who had initially found our patient and they carried with them his tattered cloth overcoat tattooed with large tire marks across the back. It seems that a truck had run over him as he lay drunk, in a heap, at a construction site in the dark.

Mercifully, I suppose, he survived. I don't know if he ever showed up in the ER again, honestly don't know if I would have recognized him among the subsequent José Does we saw in the ensuing months and years.

One thing I do know is that, now, many years later, attitudes policies, and pronouncements have coarsened and worsened and the anti-immigrant, anti-gay, anti-Semitic, anti-Black violence it has unleashed is ripping the nation to shreds. I would like to believe that more humane policies and attitudes might help to lessen the chance that other Josés would fall to the same fate as ours did if only our politicians could be exposed to the horror stories those of us, police, medics, and ER practitioners see so often. (Again, with the allegations of gang violence, pet eating, and now the extrajudicial deportations being made, what I last wrote seems hopelessly naive.)

CHAPTER 19

WHO'S IN CHARGE?

Imagine a packed ER. It's already late on a busy night. Every stretcher is full. Ambulances roll in every five minutes like clockwork. The triage nurse brings in three or four patients at a time every 15 minutes to replace the ones the Physician Assistants and I have just discharged.

Some Emergency Rooms fill up and get clogged. Patients sit, wait to be seen, wait for tests, wait to be discharged. The ER I've worked in for over 10 years is a well-oiled machine with things going so smoothly that for four years in a row, our department has won top prize in patient satisfaction in a national survey of 1200 hospitals. We have a team that has been working together, respectfully and harmoniously for several years. Nurses, PAs, aides, clerks, and physicians all overlap in their functions, understanding, and anticipating what one another needs to make sure everything gets done, and to ensure that each patient is treated correctly and with courtesy.

Unfortunately, every now and then a wrench gets thrown into the works.

"Wait a minute," I said on this particular winter night to Jen, one of the nurses I work with. She was taking care of a new patient, the man in Bed 6 whom I was about to see.

"What's the story with this guy?"

"The ambulance brought him in about 20 minutes ago. Didn't you hear their report?" She looks at me a bit anxiously.

"No. I was on Bed 8 taking care of the man with pseudo seizures," I reply.

"He was living in a shelter and just got kicked out for fighting with another resident," the aide chimes in. "He only speaks Spanish."

Fine, that's easy, I think as I walk to take this patient's history and examine him. Having spent my first two years of medical school in Mexico and then doing a residency at LA County Medical Center, I know that my Spanish is as good as anyone's.

This delusion lasts all of thirty seconds. I hadn't counted on rapid-fire Cuban schizophrenic Spanish, something I'm not fluent in. I make out individual words, and phrases about needing a place to stay, wanting to be admitted to the Psych ward, and having emotional problems. While I suddenly feel a bit off balance and not fully on top of what this man is trying to get across, I do understand enough to tell him what procedure we need to allow to get him admitted.

"That's fine," I reply to his word salvo. "We need to draw your blood. If you are depressed and want to be admitted to the hospital, we need to do routine blood tests, make sure you don't have any kind of potentially toxic drug ingestion, infection, or underlying medical problem, and then we'll admit you," I tell him.

"Esta bien," he says, nodding in agreement and we call the lab to draw blood.

He refuses to allow the lab tech near him.

I talk to him again and explain why he needs to have his blood drawn.

He nods his head, agreeing to have the blood taken.

Again, the lab comes.

Again, he refuses.

This goes on four times. Each time I am called by the nurse as I'm off tending to other patients. Each time I come back and have the same conversation.

"Look, if you want to be admitted, we need to draw your blood."

"Fine. Use this vein," he says, showing me a spot on his left forearm.

At this point, I engage Ray, a Cuban-born nurse. He approaches the patient, and I watch and listen as they verbally joust. I can see that there are philosophical, cultural, and obfuscating issues involved here but Ray can fence with the best of them. He speaks as quickly as the patient, verbally boxes him in firmly and we get another commitment for blood to be drawn.

I go off to take care of a 40-year-old man, paralyzed from the waist down from a car accident two years earlier. This is the third time I've seen him in five days. Each time he comes in with a different problem related to his paralysis. Tonight, his blood pressure is low, as is his temperature and he's dizzy. As I'm trying to work him up word comes back from Bed 6's nurse.

"Ken, he's refused again."

Ray joins me one last time at Bed 6.

"I know it's past time for you to leave," I tell Ray, "but will you tell him that if he refuses again, not only won't he be admitted but he will be escorted out of the ER?"

The information is passed on, the laboratory tech reappears, and the patient once again refuses. By this time Ray has left. I sense our ER machine is starting to lurch and clank.

Taking a break from the patient who has low blood pressure, I go to my computer to type up a discharge form for Senor Cuba, as I'm now thinking of him.

Jen goes to discharge him. Now we get the beginnings of a tirade en Espanol about how he wants to be admitted. His voice raised, I see he is escalating, upping the ante.

"Please call Security so he can be escorted out, "I tell the clerk.

The well-oiled machine is coming to a halt. I can feel the gears grinding.

I stand close by to supervise Bed 6's departure as Security approaches him. My workup on the paralyzed patient is halted once more.

This new thrust of mine elicits his new parry. He takes the discharge papers and with an accompanying Spanish tirade, leaps off the stretcher and angrily throws the papers to the floor, exhibiting flailing, aggressive body movements that tell us all to keep away.

"Please call the police," I say to the clerk, as I see that the Security guards don't want to deal with this.

We are at a standoff and the ER has been brought to a complete standstill. Nurses are watching this man now, unsure what will happen next; patients and their families are pulling open their curtains from various sides of the ER, several of them anxiously peering out; some are smiling in amusement, others are angry that their care is being delayed because of this performance.

As I turn away from Senor Cuba, I see 5 patrolmen arrive, faces grimly set in anticipation of potential violence.

I've been working with many of these cops for years, taking care of them and their families when they're sick. They also are part of the machine, helping keep it going smoothly. Some of them work part-time as paramedics and we have mutual respect and a rapport. I even get my Police Benevolent Association Get Out of Jail Free cards from them annually to keep in my car if I ever get pulled over. It's reassuring to have them arrive and I hope that their presence will allow us to get the ER moving forward again.

"Hey, doc. This guy causing problems?"

"Yeah," I say to John, the one I know the best, "He was told he had to leave if he refused to get his blood drawn. He has now refused six times. Seems like enough to me. But he's not happy with our plan and apparently, he's refusing to leave."

Five policemen, gloves on, ready for trouble, begin to surround the patient.

"What is going on here?"

I turn and see the sergeant, burly, mustachioed, now walking in.

"This guy was kicked out of a shelter; now claims he wants to be admitted...

"I don't care what happened to him. Why are you telling me this?"

I look at him in surprise. He looks pissed off.

I start again.

"He says he wants to be admitted to the Psych ward. He needs to have blood drawn if he wants to be admitted."

"So, what's the problem?" He glares at me.

"We've tried to get that done six times and each time the lab comes to draw it he refuses," I say, trying to respond as evenhandedly as I can, trying to assess what his seeming belligerence is from.

"Are you saying you're refusing to treat this patient?" he demands.

"I sense that the sergeant is now also upping the ante, for what reason I don't know. I'm saying that he understands that if he wants to be admitted he needs to have blood drawn. I can't treat him without that."

The sergeant walks away, and I watch as he begins talking to Mr. Cuba in English about what he's doing there. The machine feels as if it's actually going in reverse.

"Okay, Pancho," the cop says. "Let's see your green card."

"Ju very brave with jur gun. Jur gun and all these other guys," Mr. Cuba snarls at the sergeant.

"Right," the cop sneers.

"Ju ever use de gun? Ever kill someone?" Cuba taunts.

"Yeah, ever hear of Vietnam? Ever eat monkey on a stick?"

Cuba now looks at the sergeant wide-eyed, uncomprehending.

I have the sense that in the game of taunting one-upmanship, he's been bested. As the sergeant talks to him, I go back to my computer and watch from a distance as the scene continues to unfold. It's the sergeant's gig now.

I listen to his rants to the patrolmen about making sure it's documented that I'm refusing to treat the patient so that they're covered if anything happens when they take him outside.

It soon becomes obvious that, with the combination of the show of physical force by the police, the implied threat of deportation, and the immediate threat of being taken out of the warm ER and left somewhere on the cold wintry street, Mr. Cuba will allow his blood to be drawn. I watch as he bares his left arm, the lab tech reappears and now walks away with her tubes finally filled with blood.

As I turn to do other work on the computer the sergeant approaches me.

He stands by my side. He waits.

I continue my writing. "Fuck you, asshole" pops into my head several times.

"Doc," he finally says, belligerent tone slightly modulated down.

"Yeah?" I respond, finding myself in a new power situation after twenty ER doc years and unsure of what tone to take. "What was the problem over there?"

"Just doing what I have to do, trying to help."

"Well, it wasn't helpful to me at all. In fact, it was a drag, and I don't understand why you spoke to me like that."

The sergeant straightens up, eyebrows arch. "What are you saying to me?" he demands.

I hesitate. How far do I go with this? I'm angry and frustrated, it's 2 in the morning and I just want to get things moving again, pick up the broom, and start sweeping up again, as a colleague would say; just clean out the ER. I suddenly remember that this was the same cop who, months earlier had brought in a screaming, ranting alcoholic man, marched him to a bed and when I walked over said., "So what are you going to do with HIM doc" in a frighteningly belligerent tone.

I immediately realize that this is a dead end. If I want things to get up and running again, I need to just say, "Nothing. It's all good. Thanks for your help."

With that, I turn back to the computer, sensing that, at least for now, things might start to move forward once again.

CHAPTER 20

BANANA BAG

We sit in the quiet emergency room, tense and anxious in the silence. A couple of hours ago, the Friday night bars emptied out, and we were deluged. Our team of doctors, physician assistants and nurses were sucked into the maelstrom, forced to ride the manic energy, the rapid bursts of incoming drunken lunacy.

It's about 3:00 a.m. or 4:00 a.m. now (and the year is probably 2002) and a good thirty minutes have passed since an ambulance or police cruiser has called in on the radio. This is their standard routine, alerting the ER to be prepared, notifying us that within moments, they'll be paying us another visit, hauling in yet one more troubled soul.

In this sudden respite, we're dazed, try to kibitz a little, touch lightly on superficial topics and keep our heads down, so convinced are we that at any instant another rowdy patient will come in, shatter the calm and ramp up the volume once more.

Sure enough, out of nowhere, the ambulance doors *whoosh* open. The cops have decided to pull a fast one. Unannounced, two officers lead in a handcuffed man whom they claim is seriously intoxicated. A neighbor, frightened by the ranting he'd heard next door, had called 9-1-1 and when the police arrived at the man's apartment, they smelled alcohol on his breath. While it's certain that he will be put in jail after our evaluation, they want him to be medically cleared first.

We quickly discover the reason he needs to be incarcerated: his acute alcohol intoxication has brought out a homicidal rage, and apparently his home is loaded with guns.

"But don't worry! He's got no weapons on him now," the young, crew-cut patrolman assures us. "We made sure they were all locked up before we brought him in. You should have heard the crap he was shouting about the 'Dotheads' and 'Towelheads' he was fixin' to kill tonight. Seems like 9/11 pushed him over a bit," he adds.

The officer and his partner drop this information on us just as they are transferring him onto our stretcher and removing his handcuffs, ready to leave him in our charge. Despite the reassuring fact that he has no weapons, I observe his balled-up fists and demonic gaze as he's wheeled into a room, and I understand immediately that he has the potential to restart the chaos and inject violence into what remains of our night.

"I guess we need to get a security guard here, Officer," I say in my most ironic manner to the cop who is walking away.

"Yeah, just make sure he's white," comes back his reply, as he and his smirking partner meander out the door.

I enter the room, the brief history and the glimpse I've now had of this patient sharply etched into my brain. I take a better look: he seems to be about forty, with close, cropped dark hair, slim but muscular build, casually dressed in jeans and white T-shirt. I try to be empathic, non-threatening, careful about my body language, but I can't help being aware that he is dangerous. To my great relief, I discover that he can be pleasant.

"I'm glad they brought me to a hospital with a good white, American MD," he says with a sudden smile.

Aha! That's why he's being so reasonable, I think. *I wonder how he'd feel if he knew he had a Jew boy as his doctor.*

A few minutes later, I'm joined by Mike, the nurse assigned to this patient. I continue talking to the man, trying to get a sense of what happened before he was brought to the ER by the police. He is clearly intoxicated, occasionally slurring his words as he sits against the back of the stretcher. Mike, in the meantime, has given him a gown to put on and is checking his vital signs.

"We need to get some blood and urine from you, try to make sure your labs are all OK," I tell him, in as neutral and yet authoritative tone as I can muster.

"Yeah, well just don't get some nigger in here to draw my blood. Don't want 'em touching me," he snarls.

I ignore the comment.

"No chinks neither," he spits out.

From what we're hearing and the way he's sitting, elbows taut at his side on the stretcher, eyes constantly darting towards the door, I'm very happy when our two burly security guards saunter into the room. (Neither of them is white but our patient appears to ignore this.)

Soon he is escalating once more.

"Fucking Ayrabs. They're animals. Killed my buddies at the World Trade Center. Glad Cheney sent the troops in. After they kill those gooks in Eyeraq maybe they can drop some bombs on Israel. Goddamn Kikes started all of this shit. None of them were killed on 9/11. They got warned and never came in to work that day."

This all spews from his mouth in an incessant, drunken diatribe.

"Listen," I tell him, "I'm not interested in any of this crap. We need to make sure you don't have any medical issues and then I'm going to have the shrink see you. Decide if you need to be committed."

Mike meanwhile has gone out, gotten an IV pole, and begun to set up what we call a "Banana Bag," a salt solution mixed with vitamins. It's a treatment we frequently initiate with intoxicated patients, and the concoction has a yellowish neon tinge to it, hence its name.

He walks back into the room and calls out to me:

"Dr. Weinberg, I have the banana bag all set. Are you ready to run it in?"

"Weinberg, huh?" my patient suddenly turns his gaze on me.

"Get me another doctor," he snaps at Mike.

"Sorry, pal. You're stuck with him," Mike replies in his most nonchalant manner.

At this, the patient tries to leap from the gurney. The security guards are on him in an instant, jumping to either side of the stretcher, grabbing his arms, and wrestling him back to the bed. He starts thrashing his legs and cursing, then spitting. Mike runs out and yells to the other nurses:

"Get hard restraints, and a face mask!"

Fortunately, alerted by the commotion they'd already heard inside, several other nurses were approaching the room, and we soon have adequate help to deal with this crisis.

Two nurses grab the man above the knees as their colleagues are attaching leather manacles to his ankles. The security guards continue to hold him at the elbows as Mike starts securing his wrists. I've positioned myself at the top of the stretcher, holding his head to the side as he continues to try and spit, now at me. Forcing his head down hard, maybe harder than is necessary, I assist another nurse in getting the elastics of the face mask positioned behind his ears. The mask itself goes securely over his mouth, rendering his spittle fusillade useless as it backfires onto his face. After a frightening moment where he extricates one arm and we fight it back in, we finally have him secured. He's still writhing about, loudly rattling the stretcher he's now attached to at wrists and ankles and the wet curses continue to slaver from his mouth. But fortunately, the violence he so clearly would be happy to cause has been squelched for now.

My anger-induced adrenaline is still coursing through my blood as I wrap my tourniquet tightly around his arm above the elbow. I find a good, big vein, insert my largest bore IV just below the elbow, and tape it securely. Mike, meanwhile, wheels closer the tall IV pole, the large bright yellow banana bag and IV-line dangling from the top hook. He hands me the end of the tubing and as I attach it to the port in his forearm, my patient once again stops his anti-Semitic, anti-Muslim tirade to turn as best he can against his restraints. He seems startled by the bag and the yellow liquid that has just begun flowing into his arm.

"What's in that fucker?' he asks Mike, eyes open very wide, totally distracted by this sudden turn of events.

I turn and look him in the eye, my fury unabated.

"It's my piss!" springs to my lips.

I snap my mouth shut before the words can emerge.

But he seems to read it in my eyes.

I bring my head close and continue to stare at him. He stares back, wide-eyed and speechless, as I turn and walk out the door, grateful for the stunned silence that now engulfs the room.

CHAPTER 21

SWEET GAS

They seemed like two pixies. Just appeared at 3:00 in the morning, like rabbits coming out of a magician's hat. One moment the far side of the Emergency Room was empty and quiet, then there was a flurry of ambulances and when the smoke had cleared, we rubbed our eyes and suddenly saw two elderly women, dressed in a bright, idiosyncratic polyester style, sitting on adjoining stretchers on Bed 11.

Were they mother and daughter? Their addresses weren't the same on their charts, but they spoke in a kind of mutually understood shorthand, and they'd apparently come in together after being exposed to some "sweet-smelling" gas.

"I think it was carbon we were breathing in," the younger, more loquacious one allowed.

"Yeah, and my throat was hurting," the older one added.

They both were tiny, no more than five feet tall. And yet, as the ER began to quiet down once more, their presence loomed larger. Relaxing, plastic, oxygen cannulas astride each nostril, their ongoing, nearly delusional dialogue began filtering over to where I was sitting with the nurses.

“The Fire Department thought it was something,” the older one continued. “I mean, did you see all those guys in uniform rush in after you called them?”

“Maybe it was the white powder they left behind the oven to kill the mice; maybe when my stove got hot it started burning. Maybe that was what I smelled,” the younger one allowed.

“Yeah, I’ll bet that’s what it was,” she declared with finality when their carbon monoxide levels came back, normal as I knew they would be.

Breathing a sigh of relief, the younger one plucked the clear, pronged tubes from her nostrils, and did the same for the elder, whom she adroitly helped off the stretcher.

And then, before we knew it, and without so much as a “By your leave,” or any further explanation, they quietly disappeared back into the early morning mists.

CHAPTER 22

GINGER'S EAR

The overnight shift had been unusually quiet. So quiet that by 2:00 a.m. I'd finished seeing all the patients who'd been piling up since I'd arrived at 7:00, earlier that night. I completed all of my charts and thrilled with the thought of some well-deserved sleep, I went to lie down in the isolated on-call room behind the emergency department.

I was out as soon as I hit the pillow. Suddenly, after some unfathomable period of time, the phone rang. Strategically placed right next to my head, it wrenched me from a stupor.

"Ken, some kid just came in," Lissa, the charge nurse told me. "She's had a freaking earache since yesterday, but her mother decided that three in the morning was a good time to come in and have it checked out."

I staggered from the bed into the adjoining bathroom, threw several handfuls of cold water on my face from the sink to try to wake up, and stumbled out the door. I was semi-conscious, my head buzzing after being so abruptly yanked from sleep. As I left the room, I found myself ruminating about why I'd chosen a career that caused me to deal with so many non-crises in the middle of the night.

I rounded the corner of the Emergency Department, its stillness broken only by the sporadic and disquieting screams from the child who I realized had to be my new patient. Entering the otherwise empty, open space, I tried to focus on how I'd handle a cranky toddler with a red eardrum that was sure to be difficult to visualize.

As I picked up the chart to get more information on this patient, I realized that I first had to hide the torporous state my expressive face was sure to reveal. Always the professional, I mustered up my most cheery, concerned, and awake countenance and approached the bedside.

The remaining wisps of fog vanished abruptly as I neared my patient. She was not a toddler at all but eleven or twelve, dressed haphazardly in a dirty pink sweatshirt and baggy pants, with unkempt blonde hair sticking up from random spots on her head. And she was eyeing me with that head held at a disturbing angle.

I smiled at her, her mother, and Lissa, then directed my attention to the chart in my hand. I noted that Ginger, as I found my patient was named, had ADHD, as well as a slight fever. Looking once more at the trio, I was struck by the scowls on the faces of mother and daughter.

Mom, I observed, was a prim, tight-lipped little woman, reeking of nicotine. Her mousy brown hair was up in pink rollers, and she was dressed in a rumpled, lime-green bathrobe. And while she was probably no more than 40, I could already see the lines that nicotine had started to etch all around her mouth.

This was an entirely different scenario than I'd imagined, and I realized I had to rethink my game plan.

"Sweetie," I said, as I walked closer to Ginger. "What's bothering you tonight?"

Ginger glared at me and pointed to her right ear. "She's been complaining about pain in that ear since yesterday, but I didn't think nothin' of it till about an hour ago when she climbed into my bed screamin'," the mother professed.

I glanced first at Lissa and then at the patient. "Well, I guess we need to take a look at that ear, okay?" I asked. There was no response. Undaunted, I pulled my otoscope from the wall unit, stretched out its' long, black coiled chord as I came back to the stretcher, and showed it to Ginger. "I know you're in pain and you're probably scared of this thing, but I promise I'm going to be gentle."

Ginger and her mom continued to glare. I smiled at them again.

"If you help me and stay very still, I'll be able to see what's going on really quick." I paused. "Then mom can take you right home and you'll start feeling much better." With a barely nodded assent, she adopted a rigid pose, staring straight ahead, fists clenched at her sides in what I took to be a resignation to the inevitable.

"Hon, I'll hold your hand, okay?" her mom asked. I came closer to Ginger, black-funneled otoscope at the ready. I watched from the corner of my eye as Lissa swung into a defensive posture behind Ginger. I gently pulled down on the earlobe as I slid the otoscope in. Looking through the narrow, light-filled tube, I found the view inside the ear canal blocked by a large glob of cerumen-dried yellow earwax.

"Boy, I can't see very much," I said as I quickly pulled the scope out.

Ginger dropped back on the bed squirming. She began flexing and straightening her arms at the elbow. I took this as an ominous gesture. "You know," I said, looking first at Ginger, then at Mom, and finally, Lissa, "there's a lot of wax in there. What I need to do is rinse it out with warm water so I can see what's really causing the problem."

All three of them now scowled. I smiled in return and went to a cart that contained all the equipment I'd need. I returned with a warm water-filled kidney basin, a large syringe, and the widest bore plastic IV tip we had. At 14 gauge, "large enough to read *The New York Times* through," I knew I now had the tools that could generate a jet of water strong enough to break through the most resistant wax barricade. And done right, there'd be no damage to the eardrum behind it.

"Okay, Sweetie," I began, as I attached the soft catheter to the syringe and drew up the full 50 cc of water into it. "I'm going to gently squirt some warm water in there so that I can see what's going on."

On one side of Ginger, right next to me, was Lissa, placing a second kidney basin (to catch the water and wax as they would emerge) right under the girl's lower earlobe and an absorbent sheet on the girl's shoulder to catch any overflow.

On the other side of Ginger was her mom, tightening her grip. Both appeared ready for action.

"Here we go," I said, once again holding Ginger's earlobe with one hand to achieve the proper angle for entry, as my other hand guided the gray plastic IV nozzle into the ear canal.

I noticed Ginger's hands were clenching and unclenching, her elbows bending and unbending more rapidly. I wondered about the wisdom of my plan and whether the agony we were all about to endure was worth the inevitable endpoint: After a protracted and difficult four-person wrestling match, I'd merely confirm an infected, swollen eardrum lurking behind the wax, causing the pain, and fever.

Professionalism took the upper hand once more. Maintaining that hand became an immediate issue. As I'd feared, we were soon locked in a furious struggle. I'd squirt and retreat as the water would fly back out of the ear. Ginger would scream and twist as her mom held her with a grim determination. Lissa meanwhile had adopted a defensive pose while she held Ginger's shoulder in one hand and the kidney basin filling with murky water in the other. She was glaring at me with a look that cried out: "Why are you being so thorough?"

After several minutes of this, I stepped back to regroup, considering my options. I wondered if I should just write an antibiotic prescription and call it quits. Somehow, I realized I couldn't do that. I had to see this through to the end. With that realization, I entered an altered state. Gone were my drowsiness, and my questions about my chosen career.

Instead, I was William Carlos Williams on a late-night pediatric house call. It was Paterson, NJ in the 1930s, in the midst of a diphtheria epidemic. Concerned parents stood on either side of me as I was trying, without success, to get their adolescent daughter to open her mouth. As they watched the struggle, unable or unwilling to help, I finally used a long wooden spoon to get past her gritted teeth and hold down her tongue. I was desperately trying to look in the back of her throat to see if she had the distinctive, nasty grey membrane diagnostic of diphtheria. I thought about how often we must inflict pain and suffering to bring about a cure.

Sensing that my trio's suffering was nearing its' limits as I continued to squirt, I realized I was reaching a limit as well. I was about to give up, put my instruments down once more, and reach for my prescription pad. But then I shot a particularly well-placed bolus of water. It struck its ceruminous target at exactly the right angle and out flew a big chunk of ear gunk and the round, white plastic bead that lay behind it. They both plopped into the murky depths of the kidney basin and right before I leapt out of the way one last time, afforded me a view of the red infected ear drum that had brought her in. Ginger dropped back onto the stretcher and her mom, and Lissa, slumped over in obvious relief.

As Lissa took away the dirty kidney basin, white bead now floating on top of the foul waxy water, I walked to the ER desk and wrote a prescription for some much-needed antibiotics. And I silently gave thanks that somewhere inside me I'd been able to find a place to be persistent, do the right thing, and now could send her mother and Ginger home, well taken care of.

I know Dr. Williams would have approved.

CHAPTER 23

SHAFTED

Anytime that a nurse walks over with a smirk on their face and tells me a patient will only be seen by a man, I can pretty much rest assured that we're talking about male genital problems.

Sure enough: It was a lovely early April afternoon, a Sunday, with most people enjoying the beginnings of Spring. I had just gone out with one of my Physicians Assistants for a therapeutic "breath of fresh air," taking a psychic and physical break from a long day inside. As soon as I walked back in a nurse walked over to me, chart in hand.

"Ken, I can't wait to hear about this one." She smiled as she gave me the chart.

In the area under "Chief Complaint" was scrawled: *Injury to penis last night.*

I took the chart from her and approached the patient's room, thinking, *I know of at least one person who may not be enjoying the lovely Spring weather.*

As I entered the room I saw a young white man, in his early twenties, dressed in urban gangster style. He wore a baseball hat cocked to the side, big clunky shoes, and jeans that seemed to have a crotch that went down to his knees. He looked extremely comfortable for someone whose penis had been injured, albeit the night before.

His girlfriend, also affecting the gangster look with gaudy purple lipstick and trashy high-heeled shoes, looked at me and started to smile. "You look very familiar. Didn't you treat him two years ago when he was stabbed?"

"Hold on a minute. Was he stabbed and didn't even know it?" My mind was racing as I said these words.

"Yeah."

"And the guy who did it was let off and still lives in your town?" I asked, sensing that this would be something that they'd have no way of knowing I would know.

Now my patient spoke up. "How the hell did you know that?"

"Is your brother an asthmatic?" I threw this out, sensing it would seem as enigmatic as my last question.

"Yeah. Everyone in my family is asthmatic," he said.

"I'm not trying to seem like I have some weird psychic powers," I smiled, afraid of sounding like a putz. "Your parents brought your brother in recently when he was having an asthma attack. They recognized me and told me the whole story."

Actually, not only was the rest of the story as I was now told it, remarkable, but my involvement in the case had caused me many times to marvel over the fact this man had actually walked out of our hospital alive.

Without any prompting the young man and his girlfriend began to retell the tale (the injured penis being put on hold, as it were):

It had been a hot summer night two years earlier, at a town two or three miles from the ER where we now were. A group of nineteen and twenty-year-old kids were hanging out in the park drinking. An argument ensued and a kid my patient didn't know accosted him, getting in his face and making accusations about him and his girlfriend. Before he knew what happened this kid punched him, four or five times, in the chest and abdomen. My patient stood up and walked away, angry, but otherwise not feeling as if he'd been hurt, not wanting to strike back. When he got home, he looked at himself in the mirror and saw blood stains on his shirt over each of the spots where he'd been hit.

I had gotten involved when, about twenty minutes later, he and his friend burst through the ambulance doors of our ER.

"He was fucking stabbed!" I recall the friend saying.

"What do you mean?" I asked. Our ER was located in suburban Northern Jersey, was not a trauma center and knifing victims did not have a habit of showing up there.

As we found out, he'd been stabbed by a knife so sharp that he didn't even feel it, held in the assailant's hand in such a way that in the dark it wasn't even seen. (I was told this by the police when they came in that night to gather the evidence-that apparently never led to a conviction. They told me, after hearing the story, that they'd seen several of this type of attack before.)

We'd immediately thrown him onto a stretcher and checked his blood pressure and pulse. Blood pressure was good, but pulse was wild, racing, an ominous sign for someone stabbed in the chest and abdomen.

Not being a trauma center we had no surgeon available; I hadn't cracked a chest in years and if this kid had been stabbed in the heart, lungs, or liver (the organs directly under where his razor-thin stab marks were displaying themselves with fine red lines) he was in big trouble. Of course, an inebriated twenty-year-old kid isn't going to know about Level I or II trauma centers and what it meant to show up at the latter, late at night when the surgical team that could technically have helped him earlier in the day was long gone.

We quickly shoved in two large bore IVs, put him on the heart monitor, and got an EKG and chest X-ray while I frantically called Adolfo Zairis, our thoracic surgeon.

"Z!" I shouted as soon as I got him on the phone, "I have a kid who just walked in with multiple stab wounds to his chest and belly!"

"How are his pulse and blood pressure?" Adolfo asked.

"His heart rate is 140 but he's got a strong pulse, doesn't look shocky and his BP is 120/80."

"Get a stat CAT scan of his chest and abdomen; have them shoot in dye to look at his heart and aorta and I'll be there in 15 minutes," Z said, plunging down the receiver.

By the time Z got to the ER, the kid had gotten a liter of fluid IV, his pulse rate had slowed down to 100, and as Z and I saw on the CAT scan, miraculously neither his heart, lungs nor liver had been punctured by the non-visible knife. He was admitted to be observed overnight in the ICU and discharged the next day without any complications.

Now, here he was again, two years later, with a very different malady, a small tear on the shaft of his penis from rough sex he and his girlfriend had engaged in the night before. Luckily it was superficial enough that he didn't even need sutures, certainly not the fracture of the penis I'd worried about initially. As he tucked his Betadined penis back in and pulled up his gangster pants once more, we laughed about the interactions between his family and me, his great luck at evading any serious trauma to any of his organs so far, and he and his girlfriend went off to finally join those enjoying the lovely Spring afternoon.

CHAPTER 24

Ona Needed Me, Too

Ona called me late that afternoon from a taxi. She was sobbing uncontrollably. "I can't believe it. I just broke my foot. Again. In the same spot!"

She took a breath.

"Will you do me a favor? Call one of the orthopedists and see if he'll come to the ER at 7 when you get there for work tonight."

"Of course, O," I said. "But let's try to make it closer to 8. I never know what I'll be walking into when I get there."

I felt terrible. At the moment, I was trying to navigate the 5:30 p.m. West Side Highway traffic en route to my 7:00 p.m. ER shift and I was struck that this was the second time in three years that Ona had injured herself. She's not a klutz and doesn't have osteoporosis. What the hell had happened?

We'd been married for fifteen years at that point. Apart from the year that we met, when I was doing a very exciting fellowship in psychoneuroimmunology (looking at the interactions between body and mind that subsequently was sabotaged and inadvertently led me to the ER) I'd been working as an emergency medicine physician. In fact, it was because of this sabotage that I'd changed paths in medicine and had now been working as an assistant director of an ER in suburban New Jersey, reverse commuting thirteen times a month from our Soho loft in lower Manhattan. She and my ten-year-old daughter were familiar with the players, politics, and protocols swirling inside the hospital, having made many trips there, either on "Take Your Daughter to Work Day," picking me up (after I'd worked an overnight shift) on the way to Thanksgiving Day trips to our house Upstate, or from the times something happened in the city and it actually felt more comforting and easier, to schlep to my hospital (it was only four miles from the George Washington Bridge anyway) than to deal with the inevitable mishegoss we knew we'd encounter at any of the ERs near us in Manhattan.

So, as I'd say, familiar, but maybe not familiar enough.

At seven o'clock, I walk into the hospital. The ER doesn't seem too bad, no feeling of frenzy and I sense only a low-level intensity emanating from the nurses and PA's who are already there. Approaching my workstation, I'm surprised to come upon my wife.

"O, you're here early. How are you doing?"

"The foot looks like crap," I continue. "I'm sure you're right about it being broken. C'mon, let's get it elevated and put some ice on it."

Before I can bring over a chair for Ona to rest her foot on, the paramedic radio goes off.

"ALS 302 to Holy Name Hospital," blares the speaker.

"Go ahead," I bark into the handset, annoyed by this interruption.

"Doctor, we're five minutes out. Bringing in a cardiac arrest."

"What's the story?" I ask, wondering if this is a viable one, or just someone I'll mechanically pronounce a moment or two after they arrive.

"She's fifty-five. We don't have much of a history on her. She had a weak pulse when the ambulance got there but lost it quickly. We've been working on her for about thirty minutes, and she's just been flatline."

I run to get ice for Ona and have a nurse give her some Motrin, then hear the ambulance doors bang open and know from the accompanying sounds, that the cardiac arrest has arrived.

As I zoom back to the Code Room, watching the ambulance crew pumping the chest of this inert woman, I get more of the story.

"Yeah, she got a third epinephrine and atropine a few minutes ago, still no cardiac activity on the monitor."

"So, she's been down how long?"

"Close to forty-five minutes."

I let the crew continue a few minutes more, look at the monitor, have them stop their efforts, and watch for a rhythm on the screen. She is still flat line, asystolic, dead.

"No reason to torture her more. Let's call it at 7:33," I say, knowing anything else we do will be futile. "Any family with her?"

"Not yet," I'm told.

I run back to make sure Ona has gotten her X-ray.

"Doctor, can you come talk to the husband?" one of the nurses asks me as I approach my wife.

I take a deep breath, turn, and slowly walk back into an office next to the Code Room.

The husband is about my age, casually dressed, sitting forward expectantly. "So, how is she, doc?"

"What happened?" I ask, trying to get a sense of what he knows, what he might realize has occurred.

"Well, we were lying on the couch, watching TV and she just went out. How is she, Doc? Is she going to make it?"

I pause, looking at him. "I'm so sorry. She didn't make it. I think she probably had a cardiac arrest at your home and despite all that was done, we weren't able to bring her back."

"You're kidding." He looks at me, eyebrows arched.

Christ, I think. How in the world would I ever say that to someone as a joke? "No, I'm not," I finally say.

At this, he throws himself on the ground, screeching, wailing, pounding the floor. I find myself kneeling down, putting my hand on his shoulder, trying to comfort him.

He gradually becomes still, and silent, stands, and goes in the next room to see his wife, alive an hour ago, now dead.

I walk back to see how Ona is doing. She's sitting, leg still perched on the chair, X-ray still pending.

A nurse approaches me.

"Doctor, the son is here."

I return to the area next to the now quiet Code Room.

"Doc, what happened? How is she?"

This from the son. I look at him and try to assess what he might know. He's in his early thirties, nice face, tall, dressed somewhat gangster.

"She didn't make it," I say, holding his gaze. "We did all we could, but I suspect she had a major heart attack. By the time she got here, there was nothing we could do."

"What? I don't believe you," he says, voice rising.

"It's true. God, I wish I could say it wasn't," I barely whisper, unsure how he will react, sensing anger and rage starting to bubble up from him.

He moves forward. I back up. Then he too throws himself on the floor, wailing. He falls flat on his face, landing in the cubicle of a patient on a stretcher next to the Code Room.

Fortunately, the rest of his family, having just arrived, surrounds him, drags him out of the cubicle, stands him up, and takes him in to see his mother's body.

I remain there for a few moments, unsure what to do. After a moment, I realize I can go back to care for Ona. She's now had her X-ray and is sitting once more, waiting for the orthopedist.

By this point, the ER has escalated into shouting, beeping, phones-off-the-hook chaos all around me. The bone doctor arrives. Ona's fracture turns out to be minor. She doesn't even need a full cast. Before I know it, the car service appears for Ona, and she's gone.

The next morning, my twelve-hour shift over, I'm bleary-eyed as I drive back into the city. I'm using the one way I know to stay awake in 7:00 a.m. rush hour traffic over the George Washington Bridge back into Manhattan: Howard Stern, who I despise, on the radio. His inane rants and riffs blaring in my ear as I straggled home only to find that Ona was already off at work.

Georgia is still there, however. She greets me as she's heading out the door to walk to school. "Dad, I just want to tell you what Mom said to me when she got back last night. I know you guys have been having some issues, but she said that for all the years you've worked in the ER, she never had a sense of just how hard it is, how incredibly difficult it has to be for you to do that, to talk to families like that. I think that the screaming really got to her. No matter what you've said, how you've complained or said you were being devastated by your job, she never understood just what you must put up with."

I give Georgia a grateful hug and as she heads off to school, I go to the bedroom, throw my clothes on the floor in a heap, and drop into bed, desperate for sleep and surcease of sorrow.

CHAPTER 25

The Books They Carried

Having made writing so much a part of my career, I began to reflect on the well-acclaimed tie between writing and doctors. As a long-time emergency physician, I must and happily subscribe to Henry James's edict, "Try to be one of those on whom nothing is lost." That is the nature of medicine, particularly in the frenzy of the ER. Also, I try to keep in mind what one of my colleagues so astutely said years ago about evaluating patients in that setting,

"Always think worst-case scenario in any situation and you'll never go wrong."

Henry James, however, meant it in terms of writing. I was now seriously doing just that to help me in the ER.

Early in my career, I came upon an unusual diagnostic resource: I began noticing what my patients were reading when they showed up to be seen in the Emergency Room. This, naturally, was catalyzed by my own love of literature. But noticing what they were reading provided me some insights into their character and was a hook for beginning a dialogue on the first meeting, often in the setting of a potentially fraught medical encounter. It helped me in terms of how I should talk to them. It also allowed them to develop their own trust in me when they saw that I'd noticed what they'd chosen to bring to read when they were about to enter an unknown, perhaps life-changing, or threatening, situation. Right away, we established ourselves as person-to-person. Not doctor to illness. We created an intimacy. There was one more advantage: doing this gave me a clue into how they connected to the world, and most importantly, I realized at times it told me something about how the patient might see the story of their own illness.

I began to think about the reasons that people who are ill, or think they are, bring reading material, and what they choose to bring when they are heading off for a medical encounter. I wondered if it was random or perhaps there was something to be learned from it. Something that other practitioners could make use of.

I began to wonder if there was something on the edge there, the liminal part of an illness, an interaction between MD and patient that could be sparked by the book he or she was carrying. It was almost like a totem or voodoo doll (could a book be a new type of totem?) Do books have that much symbolism or are they trifles, just something brought along for the ride, randomly? Perhaps, because they are plugged into someone's brain already, by virtue of the connection someone develops after/as they are reading something, does that then allow a pathway in for the practitioner?

What is the connection between the books, the reading, the narrative that a patient is telling themselves and my ability to understand what is happening, what they need and to shape my ability to connect with and heal them? Is it more than just a way for me to leap into their brains as an introduction or is it deeper? What about the words or the preconscious area that the words are connected to? What happens when we get injured or are ill in those cognitive and emotional parts of our brain? It seems like, because I have gotten involved with healing and writing (as so many of my predecessors, Chekhov, Conan Doyle, Somerset Maugham, William Carlos Williams, only to name a few, have) that I'd stumbled upon something, but it often felt like I was still trying to peer over the transom at the prize(s) just behind.

Long after all these ruminations began evolving, I had left Holy Name and was working at an urgent care facility in Greenwich Village. On one of my first days there I walked into the treatment room of a patient and noticed he was reading the book, *Call me Ishmael* (words that also the opening line of *Moby Dick*. The book was the poet Charles Olson's brilliant thesis on Melville's masterpiece).

This patient, a professor at a university in New Jersey, had come in because the night before he'd spent the evening with a friend, a gay male, who had contracted meningitis. At the time, there were a number of cases of meningitis being reported in the gay community, and my patient, also gay, was concerned about his risk of contracting the disease himself. He'd come in to see whether he needed to receive the rifampin prophylaxis he'd been told could combat that risk.

"But maybe that's just a myth," he said.

"No," was my reply.

I pointed to the book he was reading. "That is a myth. Your needing meningitis prophylaxis is quite reality-based."

We both laughed, he received his rifampin, and I moved on to see my next patient. As I entered the room I was taken aback. I had to check to convince myself that the book he was reading while waiting to be seen was in fact, *Moby Dick*.

If things like this hadn't happened before I suspect I would have written this off to a coincidence, serendipity, or just to me having developed the habit years earlier, of paying attention to, and frequently commenting on, the books people bring with them. But it started me thinking more and more that there was maybe some deeper connection, perhaps synchronicity at play.

Over the years, I've had many other urgent care encounters with patients because of literary interests: I developed a long friendship with a writer, a Black woman, who was reading Philip Roth's *The Plot Against America*. When I looked surprised at her reading choice, she quipped, "He's my favorite author."

We became fast friends after that (at the time I felt the same way about Roth). I was invited to her wedding and she and her husband came to spend time with me in Old Chatham. For a year after their visit, I drove around with a copy of the book he'd left behind, *Communism and the Jews*.

Also in my short time at the Greenwich Village urgent care, I had an encounter with a patient who was reading

February House, a remarkable book about the house on Middagh Street in Brooklyn Heights that was shared in the early 1940s with, among others, Carson McCullers, W.H. Auden, Benjamin Britten, the children of Thomas Mann, Paul and Jane Bowles, and Gypsy Rose Lee. This patient was involved with a theatrical production of the story, and I was subsequently entranced by the tale of a house whose occupants' lives were inextricably intertwined and forever changed by living there, producing amazing works of art from their exposure to each other and the Brooklyn piers and bars at the end of their street. In fact, McCullers story, *The Ballad of the Sad Cafe*, was set in one of those bars, on the no longer existing Brooklyn Heights piers. Coincidentally, my cousin Joel Freeman had produced the heartbreaking film version of her book, *The Heart is a Lonely Hunter.*

Not too long before this, after 15+ years of working in several busy Emergency Departments in NYC and its suburbs, I became involved with The Program in Narrative Medicine. It couldn't have happened at a better time in my career.

My first published story, The Man Who Hugged Me, had just appeared in The Journal of Emergency Medicine (which had elicited a three-page accompanying editorial). It focused on whether we, in the ER, having only episodic, not ongoing, relationships with patients we treated there, should try to intervene/counsel certain patients when they showed up for our care due to the consequences of their self-destructive behavior.

It was around this time that I had a meeting with Oli Fein, the chair of our New York chapter of Physicians for a National Health Program. Oli, a Dean at Weill Cornell Medical School (among his many other accomplishments, he had been a White Coat Doctor in the early '60s, at great risk to himself, accompanying the Freedom Riders in the South.)

We spoke that day because, as a Dean, Oli was very thoughtful and well-versed in the options available to those of us already many years into the world of medicine. When we met, I talked about all the writing I'd been doing, and Oli told me he thought I should meet Dr. Rita Charon. She had just taken the job Oli had left in the Department of Medicine at Columbia's College of Physicians and Surgeons (P&S).

Rita, an internist, with a Ph.D. in English Literature, had started the Program in Narrative Medicine at Columbia's College of P&S recently, and Oli sensed that connecting with her could be fruitful for us both.

Rita had also thought a lot about the interface between medicine and literature, realizing that when patients developed an illness, they often told themselves a story about it. Rita had learned, as well, that when we as practitioners wrote stories about our patient encounters and shared them with our colleagues, it gave us the ability to get outside of those encounters and look at and understand them from other perspectives.

Rita and I got together right after I'd seen Oli and very quickly began to find many areas of mutual interest and passion in the world of medicine and literature.

Soon, I was involved in the program. I was teaching Narrative Medicine to the Pediatric Oncology nurses there. Also meeting several times, a month for Literature at Lunch, where a varied group of professionals from the medical school and university would meet once a week and discuss great literature, including works by Philip Roth, Bill Styron, Thomas Pynchon and not surprisingly, Henry James (Rita is a Henry James scholar).

I was invited to partake in the Adult Oncology Narrative Medicine group (which had started the whole program), where residents, fellows, nurses, and social workers would meet and bring in stories we'd written to share with and be critiqued and analyzed by the group. And I began attending Narrative Medicine Grand Rounds which occurred weekday evenings once a month. They were preceded by a lovely buffet including wine and cheese and lots of schmoozing. Then there'd be a reading led by well-known and emerging authors who had published works featuring the interface of literature and medicine, with provocative Q&As afterward.

A few years after I'd become involved, I read an article Lewis Goldfrank, of my Bellevue days, had written in one of our Emergency Medicine journals. It discussed how literature had affected his career as a physician. I reached out to Lewis and convinced him to give his own Grand Rounds at Columbia. In his typical, enthralling fashion he spoke to an appreciative, and overflowing, crowd.

Among the many things he spoke about, I most remember him showing slides of Van Gogh's work. He very convincingly (as a world-renowned toxicologist) made the case that Van

Gogh was not crazy at all, but cadmium toxic, due to his excessive use of cadmium yellow in his paintings.

It was also during this time that I was introduced to the Editor of the Science section of *The New York Times*. I submitted a story to him (which I'd read at a Grand Rounds) and which he subsequently published in the weekly "Cases" area. It concerned the events surrounding the death of my physician father.

Knowing the long and complex history of doctors as writers I feel like I've gotten deeply plugged into something, certainly something literary, but it's more than that. I began to think a lot about the connection between words and medicine, the rich, many thousand-year, multicultural language physicians have evolved to describe organs and disease processes (globus pallidus, liver flap, tic douloureux); how we grasp at words to express/convey our understanding of these bodily processes; and how, somehow, somewhere along the line, the healing we do attracts many of us to literature and writing.

Several years ago, I read a "Letter to the Editor" in *The New York Times* by an astrophysicist. He was trying to explain how his mind was constantly mulling over concepts in particle physics and quantum mechanics- but in its own language, a language that math could only try to approximate, and words barely touched.

I often wonder if the whole concept and understanding of medicine, in its own way, is like that, if I or any of my colleagues are doing the same thing as we approach a patient with a complicated disease. I certainly wrestle with understanding certain bodily processes and am entranced by the words we use to describe them. Plus, I especially enjoy bringing in Yiddishisms like *schmutz*, kvetch, and chronic *mishiganitis* to medical conversations. (In fact, one of my colleagues once remarked to me that she thought there'd be a Nobel Prize given to the doctor who could find the cure for acute *mishiganitis*!)

I am increasingly intrigued about what is actually going on in that interface of MD's brains between having a sense of what is happening with a patient and being able to articulate it and then have a healing therapeutic interaction with that person. Is there a similarity to what the physicist talked about and how does that relate to the subtle processes at play in literature and medicine, in Narrative Medicine?

As I write this, thirty-eight years after I began my first story, 22 years after I joined the Program in Narrative Medicine, I'm reminded of a trip I took in 2009 to Cambodia and Vietnam. While in Hanoi, I visited the 1000-year-old medical school there. I spent a wonderful afternoon going through the ancient buildings, getting a sense of the Vietnamese approach to illness, capped off by learning that the school was called The Palace of Wisdom. I was so enthralled by that that, the next day, sitting in the Hanoi airport, waiting to fly back to New York, I felt compelled to write about the experience to Rita. The internet was so sketchy I had just one bar on my phone. But I succeeded in having enough coverage that I was able to write Rita an email from halfway around the world, touching her deeply with the sharing of that description of the medical school.

This brings me back to the Program in Narrative Medicine. I'm a participant in a group run by my dear friend Fran, a palliative care practitioner at Columbia. I feel compelled to mention here that the week before I began attending the weekly Narrative Medicine (NM) lunches, I had met Fran and her husband, Bob, at the house of mutual friends Bella Meyer and Martin Kace. It felt like we had known each other for years as we discovered a slew of mutual connections. I probably shouldn't have been shocked then, but was when the following Wednesday, I attended my first NM lunch and found that Fran was a regular participant. I'm not sure if I should call that synchronicity or coincidence.

In the lunches, which turned into dinner meetings, we have a core circle of people whose lives and writing experiences have deeply intertwined with mine over nearly 20 years. There have been times, especially in the wake of my divorce, when I know it saved my sanity. One of the tenets of the writing is to read a story chosen by one of the members and discuss it. Then, we are each given writing prompts based on the story, and in the next fifteen to twenty minutes, each one of us writes a piece in response. It has been a fabulous experience for us all, forcing us to hone our writing skills and focus our thoughts so that often, we wind up writing a cohesive and often witty, sometimes profound, piece in a rather short time.

Other than the fact that Fran and I have been involved in this for so many years, I remember so well that one day, when we were still meeting with Rita, I'd brought in a piece I was writing ("Is Everyone Clear?") to read to the group. It was about doing CPR on a patient who'd come in awake and alert to the ER and shortly thereafter gone into ventricular fibrillation and been shocked back to life. I walked into the Narrative Writing group, and one of the nurses in the group was reading a story she'd just crafted. It too was about a patient they had recently also "coded," and been brought back, while she was at work in the ICU.

I don't know if I can characterize this as coincidence or synchronicity as well since I feel so many things that have happened to me in life sit on that fence, either because I'm open to them or maybe because I just happen to look at things that way.

What I do believe is that my involvement with literature and writing over the years has been responsible for the most profound, most important change that has occurred to me as a physician: my understanding and acceptance of the humility and total attention that I think all of us practitioners should acquire and bring to our interactions with our patients.

CHAPTER 26

STUDY OF THE PHYSICIAN AS PATIENT

"Let me put it to you this way, I wouldn't do any bike riding when you go to the country this weekend. If you fall and get a header, you could be paralyzed.'

Comforting words from the neurosurgeon. He'd just told me I had a serious problem with two of the vertebrae in my neck and needed urgent, though not emergent, surgery.

When I was given this news a little over a year ago, I'd been a physician for about 25 years, most of it spent working in the Emergency Room. I'd sent countless patients to surgery, but apart from a hernia operation at age eight, I had never had to go under the knife myself. In fact, my only medical problem is Gastroesophageal Reflux Disease (GERD), and were it not for an encounter I had two years ago with a psychiatrist, I would still be, just like many other physicians I know, without a doctor. Other than the doctor I am to myself, of course.

This psychiatrist, upon discovering that I routinely prescribed my own medication, commented that this seemed like an issue of a refusal to deal with my own vulnerabilities, getting older, my own mortality. Up until the time of this conversation, on the rare occasions when I did get sick, I had almost always taken care of myself. After all, I prided myself on my ability to diagnose and at least initiate treatment of patients with diseases across the medical/surgical/ob-gyn and psychiatric spectrum. For the occasional issue I wasn't sure about, a 'curbside' consult from one of my colleagues in the doctors' cafeteria, ER, or hospital parking lot, inevitably sufficed.

One day not too long after the conversation with the psychiatrist, and hoping to overcome my denial, I suddenly found myself embarking on a journey into new territory. I had had what I thought was just a minor medical issue and finally annoyed enough by it and realizing it wasn't going away, I buttonholed a friend who's a neurologist, in the ER.

"Mike, I've had this intermittent tingling in my left fourth and fifth fingers for about a year, and now it's become constant," I told him. He did an evaluation of me and the next thing I knew, he was leading me through a stepwise, methodical work-up. My first stop was the hand surgeon who took X-rays and did a neurological exam that was so thorough that all I could do was think about the vast amounts of pathology I was missing every day with my own patient exams in the ER. He found no pathology, however, in me.

Next, I went to a colleague of Mike's who performed nerve conduction tests and EMGs (a surprisingly uncomfortable procedure that caused my arms to flip up painfully and uncontrollably as higher and higher voltages were applied, to the muscle groups from the hand to the shoulder.) When all of this turned up nothing, I went for an MRI to, "make sure we aren't missing anything," in Mike's words.

One morning, not long after this all began, I found myself, mercifully exhausted right after a twelve-hour overnight shift in the ER, dozing off under the clanking magnet of our hospital's MRI machine.

Later that day, the radiologist (another friend) gives me the reading of my MRI.

"Kenny, I hate to tell you this, but your scan is really bad."

I was shocked. I expected it to be normal, expected that the work-up would end at this point. I listened in horror as he described a horrendous and completely bewildering degeneration of my cervical spine. Two of the bones in my neck had decayed so that, instead of the graceful C-shaped curve of a normal upper spine, mine had a sharp angulation between the fifth and sixth vertebrae (an angulation that frightened me to death when I got up the courage to look at my scan) that was pushing against my spinal cord, and had slowly, without my realizing it caused me to lose about three inches in height.

I listened aghast as he described a horrendous degeneration of my cervical spine. "You don't have any weakness or tingling?" the radiologist continues.

"No, not a thing. The only issue is the left hand," I replied.

"Well, it's funny but that part of the cord isn't really involved. The thing that is making your fingers tingle is compression on the nerve after it leaves the spinal cord.' *Ah, a radiculopathy*, I thought. So, the finger problem is just a pinched nerve.

A few days later, I spoke with a close friend and described the initial tingling that got me to the spot I was in, and she asked, "You have a *ridiculopathy*?" I laughed, thinking, *Yes, it is pretty ridiculous how I let this occur, go on so long, without any awareness of the nightmare lurking just below the surface.*

I considered this nightmare that serendipitously appeared. Did I want to know this when I began this investigation? What do I do about it? Should I have suspected something, been a better sleuth on myself? The problem that I had the MRI for was a red herring. Had I not pursued it I would never have known. Did I want to know now?

I couldn't believe what I was seeing. I was fifty-six, never sick, worked out, had great energy, and even was learning martial arts. Why didn't I see evidence of this in other parts of my body? All my bones and joints seemed to be fine. As I looked over the images with the radiologist, I was astonished: C5 and C6 had degenerated and were pushing on my spinal cord. It looked like an hourglass at that level.

How could I be moving around normally with this? I could be paralyzed if I trip or get into a tussle with a patient or horse around with my fourteen-year-old daughter, Georgia, as we still sometimes did. I was devastated. I had no symptoms but my whole self-image and approach to life changed.

I gingerly navigated New York City streets through the blizzard of '05, feeling like an old man, a walking time bomb, afraid of hitting a patch of unseen ice, falling, and not getting up. As I proceeded in the weeks before the surgery, I was more mindful of my fragility than I'd ever been and eagerly, though with increasing apprehension, awaited the scheduled procedure.

I had reasons to be apprehensive.

One night in the ER, we had a patient who was a big, belligerent, intoxicated boxer in his early twenties. The police, who had brought him in after he'd sideswiped five cars, were being uncharacteristically lax. In fact, when told his parents were coming for him, they served him his subpoena for driving while intoxicated and exited, leaving us with no security. The patient suddenly got up off his gurney to look for his hat and nearly struck the wife of a patient in the next cubicle. He then lurched toward a female nurse. Another nurse, Mike (a fairly large man), moved towards him. The tension and expectation of a confrontation electrified the whole ER. Incredibly, the patient veered off and boisterously, but without violence, left the ER with his parents trailing behind him. Once we'd all been able to exhale, Mike said: 'Gee Ken, I thought we might have a little altercation there. I was watching to see how you'd come in on it.'

I had told no one in the ER about my problem yet so I smiled and thought, *the last thing I'm going to do now is scuffle with some intoxicated boxer and become paralyzed because we're inadequately protected.*

I remembered my doctor saying, "Oh, and if you start getting any tingling on your right side, let me know at once and we'll do the surgery immediately."

I prepared to take the plunge, rearranging my schedule and notifying the appropriate people. Friends and colleagues appeared mysteriously who had the same problem and yet had decided against the surgery, giving me some moments of pause. Simultaneously, three friends told me that they were about to go in for major orthopedic surgery just as I was to have mine.

Seemingly, out of nowhere, I developed lower back pain that was more severe than anything I ever had, and I started to feel like I was having sporadic tingling on my right side. I wondered if I was somaticizing or if this was part of a phenomenon like that which happened to my wife, Ona. She was seven months pregnant and, over a period of two to three weeks, became aware that she was not feeling a lot of fetal movements. We discovered when she gave birth in a crash C-section that she was experiencing a slow, painless abruption of the placenta, and both she and my daughter nearly died in the process. Watching that process evolve, I'd subsequently come to believe that some deep, reptilian part of her brain knew all along that the placenta was trying to peel off, finally letting go of its grip when Ona was being taken down the hall to the operating room. It knew that it was finally okay, that Georgia would be safe, and therefore, it wasn't just a coincidence that as her belly was opened up, she gushed nearly half her blood volume onto the floor as the placenta tore off from the inside of her uterus.

I began to wonder if my back, and those parts of my nervous system that control balance, the posterior columns, those fancy feedback loops, my cerebellum, were all now starting to lighten up, loosen their grip in anticipation of the fact that the problem that these subliminal structures had been aware of, but that had been under the radar of my consciousness, was now going to be fixed and so I was now having these symptoms.

I went to meet my daughter after school, and as I walked up the steps of the subway, I had so much pain I could barely deal with it. Yet, when I decided to stand up straighter than I apparently had been, the pain went completely away. I wondered how I'd been holding myself for all this time, walking around with this hourglass narrowing of my spinal cord that, with the right force, could pinch off any nervous connections from my mid-chest down, causing paralysis to most of my body. How much of this was psychological?

I found myself wallowing in the fantasy of checking out, feeling sorry for myself, martyred, misunderstood. A few days before the procedure Ona and I started talking about what would happen if I died during or after surgery, insurance, finances, my wishes for her and Georgia. It all seemed surreal though as I, of course, expected nothing other than the perfect outcome to occur.

I thought about the two marathon bike rides I'd just gone on with my brothers in Florida, racing in a pack with bikers far more experienced and fit than myself, drafting each other, racing on the highway. 'Get a header' took on a whole new meaning for me.

Just prior to surgery, I needed to have a CT myelogram. I'd done more than my share of spinal taps over the years, but now the thought of a needle going into the base of my spine as the dye was injected seemed terribly daunting. I decided that I would take drugs for it. But I had a long conversation with the neuroradiologist doing the procedure and felt reassured, appropriately so. The tap was painless, and I got a perverse pleasure from watching the smoky dye track up my spinal cord on the fluoroscopy screen.

Within a few days, I had my official meeting with the neurosurgeon Michael had referred me to at Columbia. Interestingly, I'd been coming to the College for Physicians and Surgeons for the last year, to these same buildings, as a participant and instructor in the Program in Narrative Medicine. Being at the large complex of buildings at 168th Street as a 'patient' was a new and strange experience.

Although I was carrying around a low level of angst, I knew Michael held him in the highest regard and when I asked Rita (Charon) about she told me he was "the best."

I liked the doctor immediately; he gave off confidence yet displayed none of the arrogance I found so disturbing and inappropriate in many surgeons I dealt with as an ER doc. He examined me, went over my MRI and myelogram, and described all I needed to know about the operation. "Your tingling is probably going to be permanent, though," he said as he wound up the consultation. I questioned him about this. "Obviously all the exams, the EMGs, the nerve conduction tests, weren't very accurate. Look at the amount of disease you know you have yet you had normal studies." As a physician, I knew he was right, but it was disconcerting, nonetheless.

"I'm feeling quite sanguine about the surgery," I replied to all who asked. I used that word continuously until the night before surgery when I recalled that *sanguine* refers to blood; exsanguinate: to bleed out. I focused more and more on the concept of going to the other side, from diseased to well, from doctor to patient, from being in charge, running an entire emergency room for twelve hours and making all those medical decisions, to being supine, paralyzed (head bolted into place, as I find out post-op) and a breathing tube inflating my lungs as someone else takes charge and plunges into the stem of my entire nervous system. This made me think about the other meaning of crossing over—dying.

Everyone said, as a way of reassurance, that I'd be like a new man; the problem was, I hadn't known there was anything wrong with the old one.

It was the morning of the surgery, and I was sitting in pre-op. I was trying to feel calm as I looked out the window at the striking view of the George Washington Bridge and the Palisades cliffs it sits on. I was taking notes on my iBook, glad I thought to download Bach, as I find it comforting listening to *The French Suites*.

When the nurse came, I found that my blood pressure and pulse were up to 140/80 and 103. Even though I felt pretty calm my body was reacting.

I sat waiting, random thoughts going through my head. I was curious what the post-op findings would be. What day would I get home? How much pain would I be in? Would it be of a Tylenol, Naprosyn, or Vicodin ES magnitude? How about waking up in recovery after surrendering myself to The Void? We are always on the brink, but my perspective was quite different as I literally felt myself poised on the precipice.

Despite the degeneration of my spine, I still thought I had good protoplasm and wondered, as I walked into the operating room next to the anesthesiologist, how easy the recovery would be. As I lay on the table (why is it called a table? Why not something more comforting?), had the large IV placed in my arm, and felt the cool saline solution track up through my veins, I looked around the room. It looked old, big, viewing windows looking down on me. I wondered how many surgeries had been performed there. I started to panic and feel barely controlled terror. I really didn't want to lose control. These could be my last few moments alive. Fortunately, the Propofol followed the route of the saline and very quickly I was out.

It was the strangest thing but post-op I had a sense of unreality. Did I have the surgery? I felt fine before, feel fine now. Apart from the discomfort, not even pain, in my neck, I don't feel anything else, nothing feels different. And yet, I sense a feeling emerging that, being on the other side I am now fine, or will be. No more concern every time I miss my footing or drive or anticipate some kind of altercation with a patient. I find that I really don't want the morphine pump to be going, it makes me nauseous, and I'm not particularly interested in a buzz.

As I lay intermittently nodding, soft cervical collar keeping me immobile I think about how scary surgery is. Suddenly I have tremendous respect for people who need to have an operation and think especially of the patients I see who've had to come back and have it performed more than once or those with advanced cancer where there is no hope for a cure. They must go into the operating room knowing that there is no or little hope.

My recovery, recuperation, or, as I've been saying 'recouping my losses' was remarkably swift and uncomplicated. Three weeks post-surgery I went back to Columbia for the first time. I was there for pleasure, for writing, back to the prior relationship I had with the hospital. As I stood waiting for the elevator, I thought about how well the wound was healing on the back of my neck, how my relationship with it was fading, and how that parallels the distance I felt from the emotional terror I had when I came in that morning of surgery.

One year later, the tingling was still there. The scar fading. No more martial arts, but I was on my bike again, in glorious rides along the Hudson River in NYC and on the dirt roads in the mountains in Upstate New York. My scrutiny of my body, my awareness of my fragility, my mortality, was higher in my consciousness than it was before all of this and for that of others. I'd just had a patient, an obese woman who'd recently had a gastric bypass. The wounds were opening, with a liquid coming out from under the dressing that was horrible, smelling of feces. I knew she was going to be admitted, and I didn't have to do much in the ER, but I spoke to her at length, forced myself to lift the dressing to smell the wound, to know what she was going through as she lay there knowing that very soon, one more time she'd be going under the knife to a very uncertain outcome.

I'm reminded of a line from a song by Bob Dylan. "And here I sit so patiently, trying to figure out what price, you have to pay to get out of going through all these things twice." Once was more than enough.

CHAPTER 27

Korean Rice

"What do you mean, you won't transport her?" I asked, my anger starting to rise as my body tensed up and I felt my usually rational, calm self start to lose control.

"It's a state mandate, doc. If we transport that patient from your Emergency Department to a different ER, we'll lose our license."

This from a paramedic I have known for years.

"I don't care. I'll put MY license on the line. This patient is going to die. She has a freaking aneurysm of her aorta that's tearing. It looks like a water balloon leaking blood into her chest — a balloon that's going to burst at any moment and we have no capability at our hospital to do a goddamned thing to help her!"

"Doc, I just can't do it. I'm sorry."

The woman with the aneurysm had come into the ER about two hours earlier. 68 years old, petite, modestly dressed, mostly speaking Korean. None of us had any sense of what had already begun to unfold at that point.

Her husband did the translating.

They had been at home, eating Korean rice and dried fish. As she swallowed her last mouthful, she felt something strange, like a fishbone, in the back of her throat going down her chest, along her esophagus, and into her stomach. When I first saw her, she looked fine, not at all uncomfortable, blood pressure totally normal, skin color nice and pink. I looked in her throat, couldn't see any sign of a fishbone lodged there. I listened to her heart and lungs and pressed carefully on her abdomen.

Nothing about her seemed unusual. Most likely just a scratch in the throat as a bone went down when she swallowed it. But because of her age and because the husband had also said something nondescript about her having chest pain, I did blood tests, an EKG, and a chest X-ray.

They all were completely normal. When I went back in to see her, she was still lying comfortably on the stretcher.

At this point, I was ready to discharge her. It seemed the typical story of someone who had probably swallowed a fish bone, was in no apparent danger, and needed follow-up as an outpatient. As a courtesy I called her private doctor, and told him the situation, hoping to arrange for him to see her the next day.

Instead, he asked that I contact the ENT doc on call, have him come in to see her and if needed, use the thin, little black endoscope he could slide through her nose and down her throat to see if she still had a foreign body stuck there.

This seemed like a reasonable request. While I had had issues with this particular ENT doctor not responding to his pages in the past, the ER wasn't too busy on this Sunday afternoon and I was feeling optimistic, so we placed a call to the specialist. I figured if he didn't call back within an hour or so, I'd discharge the woman. Putting this situation in a compartment toward the back of my brain, I went on to see my next patients.

As I should have anticipated for a late Sunday afternoon, the ER exploded. Within a half hour, I had several sick patients requiring my attention, including an unfortunate alcoholic woman in her forties, back with us for the second time in two weeks for recurring delirium tremens, and a man in his fifties who was brought in by ambulance from the train station. He had had cardiac bypass surgery a few weeks earlier, had Hepatitis B and C, was on blood thinners and since he had gotten on the train from Manhattan to visit his mother in New Jersey, he had been passing bloody stools. (I must confess that, in addition, I had a third-year medical student shadowing me that day as well. Each time we had a moment, she and I and one of my more conservative ER partners were sporadically debating the pros and cons of national health care and how our nation's lack of Universal Coverage was impacting each incoming patient's care.)

All of this had caused me to forget about my patient with the fishbone, until suddenly, the nurse taking care of her yelled out:

"Ken, the patient in Bed 26 just became clammy and her blood pressure dropped to 60!"

According to her nurse, up until that point the patient had been sitting in a comfortable silence, patiently waiting for the ENT doctor (who, despite repeated tries never called back). Then in an instant, she had lost all her color and slumped back, nearly passing out.

I rushed in to find her lying on her stretcher, her feet now placed higher than her head in an attempt to bring blood back into her heart and brain. There was a nurse at either arm frantically putting in IV lines and running fluids in the hopes of raising her BP.

The husband was just off to the side of the bed, mouth open, clearly not comprehending what had just occurred. His wife looked terrible, ashen, covered in sweat, and barely conscious.

As I desperately tried to figure out what had just caused this and what the connection was between her throat discomfort and the sudden crash, I was reminded of another patient from not long before, a middle-aged man who also had come in with throat discomfort. Before we could try to figure it out, he had died of what we later learned had been a ruptured aortic aneurysm.

I immediately ordered a CT scan of my patient's aorta. The fluids she was getting through her IV lines brought her pressure up, she seemed to stabilize, and we rushed her over for the scan. In less than ten minutes, I had a call from the radiologist.

"Kenny, look at the scout film on the CAT scan of her chest. I can't believe it. I read her chest X-ray an hour ago and it was normal. Now, her whole chest cavity is filled with blood! She has a dissection of her aorta just where it leaves the heart and she's leaking blood into her chest!"

I called the cardiothoracic surgeon. My patient needed to go to the operating room ASAP.

He called me back within minutes. But when I told him about the reading from the CT scan, he told me that our hospital wasn't equipped to do this type of emergency surgery. She would have to be transferred to a hospital ten minutes away. Fortunately, her blood pressure remained stable. She'd gotten her color back and looked remarkably well, especially for someone whose aorta was tearing and leaking. I called the medics to arrange for transport but strangely, no one answered despite my trying them several times.

The patient was critical, needed immediate transport and was just sitting in our ER in a situation where we were useless to her. Already anxious, I quickly became frustrated and angry. I had no idea why the medics weren't picking up their phone but since their office sat right next to the ER, I ran out to their building.

That was when I had my confrontation. All I had in my mind at that moment was an image of my patient's aorta, blood oozing from it into her chest each time her heart beat. I was getting out of control, desperate to have her transferred. I was afraid she was going to bleed out and die in my ER before she was able to get the chance to have the intervention she needed.

Realizing that nothing would move the paramedics to break the rules, afraid I was going to say or do something I would regret as I stood, furious in front of them, I went to a higher authority. Picking up their office phone, I reached out to the on-call administrator of the hospital and quickly told her the situation. She leaned hard on the medics, and told them she'd take responsibility, and they relented.

Within minutes my patient, miraculously still alive, awake and alert, was being transported out of our ER. On the stretcher next to her was the CD containing all her critically needed CT images. I felt like I could finally take a breath, refocus and start wrapping up loose ends as my twelve-hour shift was just about to end.

As I started to tell my incoming partner about the patients still needing workups, I got a frantic call from the surgeon at the other hospital.

"Ken, the CD you sent isn't compatible with our computer. The patient is on the OR table now and we can't proceed!"

Shifting gears once more, I quickly got our CT tech on the phone, explained the situation, and called the local police department. As I prepared to walk out the door, I saw flashing lights and heard police sirens blaring. The cops ran in, were handed a large envelope and quickly zoomed off into the night, carrying the reformatted, compatible CD.

I drove home feeling frazzled and frustrated. The last few hours, with the patient crashing, the legal roadblocks preventing the medics from taking her; the technological incompatibilities preventing her from starting her surgery as she lay waiting in the operating room; our unbelievable good fortune that in the frantic swirl of the late afternoon I'd forgotten about the ENT doctor so that I had never discharged the patient home; and my own, sudden realization that her "fishbone" had not been that at all, filled my head on the drive. That all tended to distract me from thinking about how slim her chances were of getting off the operating room table alive.

The following morning, I had to get up early. I had an 8:00 a.m. flight to visit my daughter at college. As I sat on the plane waiting at the gate, I called the ER and spoke to the charge nurse. He told me he had just heard that my patient from the night before had miraculously made it out of surgery alive and was now in the ICU, stable.

One week later, after returning home from my visit, I was back in the ER again, events swirling around me once more. Amid that day's madness, an elderly Asian man approached and introduced himself. It was my "fishbone" patient's husband. He had just that morning taken his wife home and had driven by the ER on the off chance that I was there.

He smiled.

As I shook his hand and smiled gratefully in return, I thought back on how different things might have been and how I'd never think of Korean rice and fish in quite the same way.

CHAPTER 28

When Harry Met Kenny

Harry had been a regular fixture at the hospital a lot longer than Kenny had. But, unlike Kenny, Harry was not an MD.

He was a patient, a "frequent flyer," with serious, recurring, psychiatric and medical problems. These issues had been bringing him to the hospital long before Kenny's arrival as a full-time attending physician in the Emergency Department.

While no one ever seemed to know what would cause these problems to randomly erupt, Kenny quickly learned that every so often, inevitably at 2 or 3 in the morning, Harry would put in a call from the pay phone at Louie's Charcoal Pit, down the block from the ER where Kenny worked.

One of the nurses would answer the call and soon be sucked into a circular, exasperating, chaotic, and interminable, conversation. There would be repetitive responses and frequent eyebrow-raising looks on the nurse's face. Those of us working nearby and now unwittingly engaged, powerless to turn away, would find ourselves listening, knowing exactly with whom the nurse was conversing and that the dialogue would inevitably end with the comment:

"Harry, all I can say at this point is, even if you are over an hour away since this is bothering you so much you should come in and be evaluated by the physician now."

Sure enough, within minutes, straight from his phone booth/office at Louie's, Harry would miraculously appear. His arrival was always preceded by the sounds of his garrulous voice, wafting through the open windows separating the Triage Office from the main Emergency Department.

Harry would be expostulating about the latest medical tragedy about to befall him, and nearly without fail (despite the explicit posted regulation preventing non-hospital personnel direct access into the ER) he would burst through the doors from Triage right into the cavernous main room of the Emergency Department.

He'd always be clad in his creatively mismatched clothes, combinations of plaids and stripes, and his ratty, matted down brown hair and smudged thick glasses, perilously perched on his nose, would be virtually unchanged from his last visit.

Affecting a right or left-sided limp, according to a calculus never revealed, he'd stagger into the ER and plant himself in front of the aforementioned nurse's station, ready to begin his latest routine.

Somehow, always aware of his presence no matter where I was or what I was doing, I knew I had to steel myself for the inevitable.

"Hey, KENNY!" he'd shout, a big smile on his face, drawing out the NNY in my name, as if to emphasize his great affection for me and our deep, ongoing friendship.

This scenario had repeated itself for many years, often to my chagrin and more often, to the amusement of the nurses and orderlies who always seemed to be standing around when he'd appear.

Even though he was unkempt, unwashed, and frequently delusional, Harry was a funny and engaging presence. He rarely actually registered as a patient but would usually just plop himself down, uninvited, on one side of the large nursing station table and begin rambling, going from one topic to another randomly. If it wasn't a busy night, most of the nurses and orderlies would join him. Even the younger, newer nursing students, while put off initially by his bizarre appearance, fetor, and presence, would go from watching at a distance to sitting down and eventually joining in as his tirade proceeded. With his big grin and easy manner, mixed with the piercing observations so many psychotic patients seem to be able to pluck from the ether, it was hard not to warm up to him and join in the banter.

As I was usually busy our interactions were typically brief:

Harry: "I can't pee. Is that a blockage?"

Me: "How long has this been going on?"

Harry: "About 3 weeks. (pauses) I don't want to go to no urinologist!"

OR-

Harry (standing and eating a Baby Ruth): "I want my cholesterol checked."

OR-

Harry (dressed on this occasion in checked shirt, brown corduroy sports jacket and thick, soiled mismatched tie): "I've been suffering and it's accelerating over the last 31 years, 2 months, 3 days and (checking his watch) 2 hours and 10 minutes."

Followed by:

"I'm watching my destruction; I'm watching my mother's obliteration."

Then:

"I'm leaving."

And out the sliding ambulance doors he'd go.

Unfortunately, the last time we all saw him, we encountered another Harry.

His arrival was still preceded by its telephonic announcement from Louie's, and he was still in his usual unkempt, nicotine-odored attire when he appeared. Unlike the dozens of previous visits where his behavior seemed so benign, even when it was clear that he had plunged deep into the morass of his schizophrenic delusions, something had changed this time.

Of course, this particular Friday night, the ER had already been tilted towards psychosis and psychic despair anyway. There'd been a fight at one of the local bars, and several of its former patrons now occupied stretchers in the ER. They were in various stages of alcohol intoxication, challenging us with their many disturbing and exuberant drunken displays.

Two had minor head injuries, including a twenty-year-old woman with a laceration through her right ear. Dina, my physician's assistant, was in the process of sewing that up.

Another patient, not intoxicated, had just come in, under arrest. The police who brought him told us that when they had started booking him, he'd claimed that not getting his Thorazine would cause his nose to bleed. Skeptics that they were they locked him up anyway. Now he was in the ER, having made believers of them when, as soon as he was put into his cell, his nose had begun to drip blood. He'd been brought in and placed sitting forward on a stretcher, blowing crimson clots from both nostrils into a large plastic basin.

And just to ensure he'd have a longer stay, he'd decided to tell us, as soon as we did his evaluation, that he was also suicidal and homicidal.

By the time Harry made his entrance, this patient was still sitting on a stretcher at one side of the ER, his nosebleed having spontaneously and miraculously resolved. He was now handcuffed and being watched over by a young, nondescript police officer whose presence I'd barely noted up till then.

That all changed when Harry appeared. As I said, something was a bit different with Harry this night. He saw me as soon as he barged in. I was across the room treating a patient with bad asthma. She was still wheezing despite several hours of our intense ministrations.

Harry became offended that I wasn't immediately available to minister to him instead. So, with his usual voluble, hypomanic voice and outlandish behavior much in evidence, he strode towards me.

As I turned to chastise him for disrupting the decorum of the ER, he yelled out: "That's all right! You keep away from me. I don't want no Jew doctor taking care of me tonight anyway."

Knowing Harry's mishegoss and mood swings as I did, my first reaction was to laugh this off. Out of the corner of my eye, though, I watched as the cop, who'd originally seemed so anonymous and nondescript to me, stand up and suddenly spring to life. Moving away from his psychotic, suicidal (formerly nose-bleeding) prisoner, he quickly strode toward Harry. I immediately realized that the cop was probably Jewish, and I saw that he appeared deeply offended by this comment.

Looking beyond the officer, I saw that he wasn't the only one now engaged. Two of the nurses and an aide, sensing the volatility of the moment, were moving towards Harry as well, their eyebrows raised, mouths open, yet unable to speak.

Harry himself was taken aback. He seemed surprised and perhaps even disturbed at what had come out of his mouth and its obvious effect on everyone around him. But never one to look a gift horse in the mouth, he now added a new element to his repertoire. Despite having come in for an alleged abscess in a tooth, he decided to bring out another exhibit from his multifactorial disease inventory. As the cop and I converged on him, for very different reasons, he began to cough.

It wasn't a cough to be taken lightly. It wasn't even one of your run-of-the-mill hacking coughs, brought out in certain social situations to clear the air or make a point. Not a short cough at the end of a maneuver to clear the throat and bring up a discreet bit of phlegm or saliva. This was a fusillade of a cough, wet, prolonged, and designed to empty the lung bases of weeks of diseased and putrefying tissue. A cough that is, that was so offensive, unexpected and rude that, even had it not been produced only a few feet from where I was now standing, would have been sure to cause a startled reaction from even a seasoned professional like myself.

As our group of medical and law enforcement professionals stood, unsure how to proceed, Harry now went off on a psychotic verbal rant, interrupted increasingly by paroxysms of more disturbing coughs.

After another round of worsening coughs and wheezes, Harry collapsed on the ER floor. The assembled group scooped him up from in front of the nurses' station and gently but rapidly lifted him onto a nearby stretcher.

We quickly began giving him breathing treatments. And while we stabilized and then admitted him, for some strange reason, I never saw Harry in our ER again.

CHAPTER 29

Is Everyone Clear?

It was a ghastly Friday afternoon.

The phone lines scattered throughout the Emergency Room were ringing in a staggered, incessant, staccato succession.

The ringing was accompanied by the sounds of the pneumatic tubes, whooshing and clunking as they transported their vital cargo of drugs, blood, and other bodily fluids between the ER and the vast, multifarious network in the hospital's core.

All the institution's beds were filled, and patients had been piling up in the ER for days. Every treatment slot was now holding two stretchers in a space normally allotted for one. Each of the local ambulance crews had been notified that it would be unsafe to bring us anyone new...

Suddenly, during this madness, the medic radio sputtered and beeped: "Park Ridge Ambulance. Park Ridge. We're en route to your facility..."

Maggie, one of our savvy nursing aides, raced to the console. Though still in her early twenties, she'd already become seasoned and cynical. Scowling, she snapped into the handset, "This ER is on bypass. I called you myself an hour ago."

"Park Ridge ambulance coming in with a fifty-year-old male with chest pain," they continued.

"Don't bring him here!" Maggie shot back.

"We're two minutes out from your location," they intoned, and then the radio went dead.

Two minutes was an exaggeration. Almost before Maggie slammed down the receiver the ambulance doors whooshed open and accompanied by the sound of stretcher wheels clicking and walkie-talkies squawking, the crew rolled our new arrival in. Not having a defined place to go, they parked themselves, and their charge, in the middle of the ER's cramped open space between the nursing station and treatment slots.

The patient they brought was a gray-haired, overweight man, mid-fifties, his long legs extending past the end of the gurney. Perspiration glistened on his pale round face and dark lines traced the V of a widening triangle of sweat across his white, button-down dress shirt.

While his eyes seemed calm and detached as they stared off into the distance, his sense of dread was evident in the tight set of his mouth and jaw as he lay braced against the back of the stretcher. I turned to get a sense of his condition and was struck with the thought that he seemed like an island of impending disaster in the middle of the ER sea, as nurses, lab techs and wheel-chaired patients eddied around him.

"Here's the guy with the chest pain. Vital signs are stable..." the crew began.

"You're going to have to wait RIGHT there," the charge nurse growled, cutting them off, "until we can figure out where to put him!"

So, there they stayed, two self-conscious EMTs, shifting uneasily in their thick, black leather utility boots, and their patient, hair now matted with sweat, eyes frantically darting around as he looked for any opening of the curtains that would reveal an available bed, a safe place to moor.

Finally, a place was made for him in Slot Six and the ambulance crew gratefully wheeled him over. The nurse who ordinarily would have overseen this man was on Bed Seven tending to a frightened, wheezing four-year-old, so Maggie and I went to assist the two EMTs. I helped lift the patient onto the hospital gurney, taking the opportunity to look closer at him and feel for his pulse. It was not as strong as I would have liked.

Maggie, despite years of EMT and ER experience, would never have been left alone with this man had there been any nurses available. As there were none, she reached into a drawer in the nightstand against the wall and handed the man a gown.

"I need you to lay down so I can do an EKG on you," she said, her voice uneasy.

At that moment, I was pulled away by the conversation I overheard on Bed Seven.

"Please, Josh! You need to keep that mask on your face!" the nurse was saying. Her crisp, barely controlled tones told me that this child might be about to crash, and I strode to Bed Seven as Maggie closed the curtain on Bed 6 behind me.

I'd barely had a chance to reassure myself that the asthmatic was relatively stable when Maggie screamed, "*Dr. Weinberg!*"

I raced back to Six, tore open the curtain, and saw her bending over our new patient. He was now flat on his back, inert, not breathing. The EKG machine, its twelve grey electrical cables, and their red leads, were now barely attached through the sweat on his chest, arms, and legs. Foot after foot of tracing paper was spewing from the side of the machine onto the floor. The lines being traced showed Ventricular Fibrillation, a pattern of erratic and random electrical activity corresponding to the random and ineffectual muscle twitching that was clearly occurring in our patient's heart. The only way to bring him back to life was to shock or defibrillate him.

"Where's the freaking Code Cart?" I yelled.

"Right behind you. I'm charging the defibrillator now!" Maggie cried as she wheeled the cart in, while simultaneously shouting out:

"There's a Code on Bed Six!" The machine began the crescendo of its familiar, high-pitched whine as I ripped the paddles from it. Applying them to his chest I watched the electrical joules on its red-numbered display shoot up from 0 to 200 and heard the whine transformed into an insistent beeping, notifying us that it was ready to deliver its charge.

I shouted to all involved (making sure that no one else would be hit by the shock I was about to administer): "Everybody Clear?" I squeezed the buttons on the paddles. The jolt shot through him and his large body convulsed, a huge wave cresting and crashing, the undulation flowing up to his head and then receding down to his feet.

I turned to look at the monitor, to see if he needed another shock. One of the nurses felt for a pulse. As I turned back to the patient I watched as the first convulsion was abruptly followed by a second paroxysm and then a third. I'd never seen this before and I immediately sensed that we were witnessing a struggle occurring not just on a physical, but on a psychic plane as well, as if his soul was being torn between life on Earth and the Hereafter. The patient began moaning maniacally, his eyelids flickering before a lifeless gaze, as his massive body thrashed from side to side. The moan soared into a scream as his arms and legs shot out randomly in all directions. Maggie, the five other people from the Cardiac Arrest team, and I all pounced on him, grabbing any body part that we could to prevent him from flipping onto the floor.

Now, locked in a furious struggle, we all were slammed against the metal bed rails, the mattress, and the wall behind him. As we tightened our grips, anticipating a protracted brutal onslaught, his shrieking abruptly dropped to a whimper and his writhing stopped; his eyelids opened, he took in deep breaths, and began to look around at all of us.

Feeling him come fully back to life the team slowly eased off. I allowed myself a deep breath, and all I could think was, 'My God! He was going into the White Light, and we just snapped him back here like one of those red rubber balls attached by elastic string to a paddle.'

Within minutes he began talking and acting like nothing had happened. And while this event had profoundly rattled me, the ER was so busy that I never had a chance to go back to talk with him about what he, and the rest of us, had just gone through.

Instead, I immediately notified the cardiologist on call to admit him to the CCU and we all plunged once more into myriad other tasks we'd been doing before.

The patient remained stable for the rest of my shift until he was transferred out of the ER, and I went home that night and recorded all the details of the event I could remember.

About a year later, I ran into Maggie in the hospital. She had subsequently left the medical field and had come back to pay us a visit. I sat down to talk with her and told her I'd written a story in which she played a pivotal role. She gave me a curious smile, right eyebrow raised ever so slightly. "Do you remember one horrible, busy Friday afternoon that you were working, a guy came into bed 6, you went to do an EKG on him, and he went into cardiac arrest?"

"Oh my God! Of course, I remember." She paused.

"I'll never forget that day. As soon as I laid him down and put the leads on him to do his EKG, he stopped breathing. There was a nursing supervisor close by and she told me to pound him on the chest to try to get his heart started again. Of course, it didn't do a damn thing and that's when I screamed for you."

I smiled, hearing her experience of the event.

She stopped for a moment and then continued: "You know what that bastard said to me, after we resuscitated him and I was getting him into a gown, drying him off, completely freaked about what had happened?"

She looked at me for a response. I shook my head. "So, not only was he pissed that he thought my laying him flat had caused him to stop breathing but he said, 'You know, I was on my way out, saw my body from above. I felt myself going somewhere so peaceful and calm after that last hour of panic and pain, and you yanked me back!"

I thought again of that moment when it had been so clear to me that this man had come back from beyond. I remembered the drama, the abrupt change as his inert, flaccid body seemed to re-inflate with life. I had thought, until Maggie and I had this conversation, that someone coming back from the dead would be ecstatic to be alive, so grateful and generous to those who'd saved him, but at that moment I realized that maybe it's just from this side of the Great Divide that we value life above all else; from the other side, it isn't like that at all. Maybe that's why he'd been so nasty to Maggie. Having seen what the Hindus call Maya, or illusion, from over there, he was angry at us not only for "killing" him but for bringing him back here as well.

CHAPTER 30

CRYING

The light on the radio console started flashing a moment before its insistent, electronic, "Whoosh...whoosh...whoosh" whipped through the air, overwhelming the background clamor of the noisy ER, alerting us that the medics were calling about an incoming patient.

I hate the sound and frequently find myself wanting to rip the handset out of the console as I run to pick it up.

"Go ahead!" I shouted into it before the medics even had a chance to say a word.

"Dr. Weinberg, we're en route to your location. We have a 54-year-old woman with chest pain. EKG looks like an acute MI."

"Is she still having chest pain?"

"Yes."

"What's your ETA?"

"We're five minutes out."

I hung up and turned towards Terry, the charge nurse. She'd clearly heard the electronic alert as well, and before I could utter a word, she glared at me, eyes wide.

"What are they bringing in NOW!?!" she pleaded, frustration and vulnerability scrawled across her face.

Although the 7 PM night shift had barely started, things were already veering out of control.

"Chest pain, abnormal EKG. It could be real. If she's having a heart attack, she's a candidate for the new angioplasty protocol. Sounds like you should notify the cardiac cath team and find out which doctor is on call for interventional cardiology. They should know they may need to get here right away."

A few moments later, I heard the ER doors sliding open and watched the patient get wheeled in. She was balled up on the stretcher, her moans of pain muffled as they seeped out through the oxygen mask covering her face.

"How are her vitals?" I asked the medics as they came into view.

"Her blood pressure is holding at 105. Her heart rate is 60."

I immediately followed them to the bedside as she was transferred onto our gurney and started to talk to the patient, annoyed that there were already six other people hovering over her: nurses, registrar, EKG tech, and ambulance crew.

Despite my urgent need to get her history and examine her, I attempted to be understanding. Everyone was trying to get her plugged in, putting everything in place so that, if she met criteria, she could get her MI (Myocardial Infarction or heart attack) treated by one of our cardiologists who'd been recently trained in therapeutic cardiac catheterization. It was a technique that involved threading a special catheter into the arteries supplying the heart. Once the catheter was in, they could inject dye to identify any blockage in one or more of those arteries and immediately open that up. They'd then put in a stent, keeping the artery open and allowing vital blood flow back through that artery into the heart. If done quickly enough studies showed that this procedure could prevent permanent damage to the heart.

Up until this point, Emergency Medicine guidelines and hospital policy had my ER colleagues and I following a different protocol: We'd inject a clot-dissolving medicine into a vein in the arm of MI patients immediately upon arrival. This earlier technique had been the gold standard for opening up the clogged arteries causing a sudden heart attack, with what had been considered very good results.

Recent studies showed that the cath results were even better, but the issue was that the findings mandated that these new patients had to get into a Cath Lab in under 60 minutes from the time they arrived at our door, otherwise, they wouldn't be eligible for the treatment.

In addition, the Emergency Medicine and Cardiology staff had been told that if we accumulated enough of these new patients, we would show the State of New Jersey that we were ready to be accredited as a Chest Pain Center, bringing big money and prestige to the hospital.

What it meant for the ER staff, however, was that we could potentially be forced to stand by for an hour, waiting for the cardiologist and Cath team to arrive. If they didn't, and the allotted time passed, we were then finally allowed to inject the clot-dissolving medicine. And the problem was, though the outcome with caths was better, we could all be faced with a fraught, perilous hour, clock ticking, with a patient in pain, having a heart attack, at great risk of sudden death. We no longer could immediately and definitively treat but could only stabilize, as we waited for the specially trained cardiologist to arrive.

The stress on everyone was intense. We needed (and felt great pressure from the administration on this) to show that our medium-sized community hospital was now State of the Art, adding a whole other dimension to the stress we already felt anytime an MI patient appeared.

"Did you take an aspirin?" I asked, pulling the mask away from the patient's face.

She was a young-looking Hispanic woman, dressed casually in jeans and a work shirt.

"Yes, just before I called the ambulance," she whispered, looking me in the eye, discomfort twisting her features.

I glanced over at Terry.

"Have we reached the interventional cardiologist?" I asked.

"Well, we did reach his partner, but he doesn't do caths."

"They have no one else around? Those guys are supposed to be available immediately, ready to be here in ten minutes."

Terry shook her head in annoyance.

"Goddamnit!" I muttered. "Let's try the second cardiology group."

As we were talking, Antonio, the patient's nurse, placed a nitroglycerin tablet under her tongue for her ongoing pain.

"Ken," he called out a few moments later, "her pain's still at a 10 and her pressure just dropped."

"Squirt 200 cc of saline into her IV," I said, twisting to face him. "Hopefully that'll bring it up."

The fluids shot her blood pressure back to a safe level and I turned, shouting to Terry. "Did we get anyone yet? How about the cath team? Are they on their way?"

She scowled. It had been fifteen minutes since the patient had arrived. She still had no relief from her pain.

I left her bedside and walked over to Terry.

"Please, page them all again."

"This is the third cardiologist in that group we're trying," she answered.

"This is not the way this is supposed to go down. Have the operator call them at home then," I said.

I went back to my patient. She was moaning, still very uncomfortable. Despite more nitroglycerin, we had only been able to get her pain to a 7 out of 10.

I gently took her hand; she squeezed mine hard in response.

Again, I yelled to Terry: "No callbacks yet?" Her grimace told me no. I felt angry, stymied, and powerless, realized my hand was now squeezing the patient's as hard as she was mine.

"Try another cardiology group!" I hollered, starting to feel like I was losing control.

It was now thirty minutes since she'd arrived, and her pain was only down to a 6.

All I could think was that the number 6 meant she was still having a heart attack as I stood there. My anger now turned to fury as I was struck with the thought that if we weren't trying to become a Chest Pain Center, I would have injected the clot buster medication into her vein twenty-five minutes earlier and probably saved her, and all of us, this pain and anguish.

I continued holding her hand trying to at least transmit love and healing into her. I found myself imagining the muscle fibers in her heart, deprived of blood and oxygen, dying. Then as I stood there fuming, the last cardiologist available called back.

"I'm eating dinner," he said when I ran to the phone. "I'm not on call. Where are all the other docs?"

"No one is around, no one is calling back. She's having a freaking heart attack and I'm standing here feeling like a totally ineffectual putz!"

"Okay. I can be there in fifteen minutes or so," he told me, the irritation bristling in his voice.

I raced back to the bedside; her BP had dropped again despite more fluids. Through it all her pain was unrelenting. I stood with her and took her hand again. I didn't know what else to do.

"Ken, the cardiologist wants to talk to you again," Terry said, her own frustration evident in the curtness of her tone.

I dropped my patient's hand and dashed back to the phone.

"Hi. Are you on your way?" I asked.

"Yeah, but I just wanted to ask you a question, not that it really matters."

He paused and I realized he was probably swallowing his last bite.

"Does she have insurance?"

I held my tongue, afraid of screaming at him and making him turn and head back to dinner. I picked up the chart and glanced down at it. I rarely look at whether or not someone has insurance, so I didn't know.

"Medicaid," I told him and hung up before he could respond.

I raced back to the patient. She was sweating and then the heart monitor showed a dangerous, but momentary, slowing of her heart rate, pushing me ever closer to my own brink.

Mercifully the slowing appeared to resolve spontaneously, and the cardiologist called again.

"Tell the cath team to meet me up in the lab. I'm 5 minutes away," he announced.

I relayed this to Terry.

"The cath team isn't here yet," she tossed out, irony clear in her tone.

"When can I give the goddamned clot-buster?"

"She still has 10 more minutes to get to the cath lab."

Her heart rate dropped to 40.

"She's gonna crap out," Antonio whispered to me. "She's gonna die before we get her there."

We pushed more medications, and her rate went back up. I was still holding her hand. I started to stroke her brow as well. My frustration was overwhelming.

Another thought seared through my brain: 'We should just put in a call to the fucking priest!'

It was now 58 minutes.

"OK," Terry announced, "the cath team is ready. Let's take her up."

Everyone gratefully shifted gears. The patient was wheeled out of her slot, Antonio pushing the stretcher from behind, heart monitor beeping at her feet, aides arrayed around the bed holding the numerous I.V.s, pumps, and paraphernalia.

As she sped past, I leaned over and told her everything was going to be fine.

I didn't believe it.

For the next hour, I was agitated, infuriated. As much as I tried to stay focused on the new patients, I found my thoughts going back to all that had just occurred.

Just then, Antonio came back down, a huge smile on his face.

"Ken-She did great! He got in immediately and saw her right coronary artery was totally blocked by a clot. He opened the blockage, put in a stent and you could see the dye go all the way through the vessel where the clot had been. She's in the ICU, doing fine."

As I heard this, I felt a sudden lightness. My focus returned, and I finished my shift with newfound energy and elation. I went home first thing the next morning, slept deeply till midafternoon, and that night was back in the ER once more.

When I arrived, Elston, the lab tech who'd been involved in drawing blood from my patient from the day before, immediately walked over to me.

"Ken, I just saw her in the ICU. She's doing really great!"

I didn't need to ask whom he meant, and I immediately realized I'd have to go to the Unit, something I do so rarely that I had to be reminded where it was.

I walked into that busy setting and saw her through the glass in her room with her nurse, Karen. I entered and the patient, now resting comfortably, turned to me.

"I was just thinking about you," she said, smiling.

"How are you feeling?" I asked, smiling back.

"I'm fine. Thank you so, so much."

I approached, held her hand once more, and wanting Karen to know why I was there, but concerned that the patient would learn about how close we'd all come to disaster, I gave an edited version of what had occurred the day before.

Karen listened, smiled at us both, and then left the room.

As she walked out, I suddenly felt overwhelmed.

I bent and gave my patient a hug. Unexpectedly, all my emotions, bottled up from the night before, burst out, and tears came to my eyes.

My patient squeezed me in return, and we sat and sobbed together, each for our own reason, acknowledging to each other how deeply felt and literally heartrending those 58 minutes the day before had been.

CHAPTER 31

FIRING FROM HOLY NAME

After twenty-two years, tumultuous as they often were, I was unceremoniously fired from Holy Name. The ER contract was up for renewal, and I was told that the Administration would not renew it unless I was given the heave-ho. It was unclear if the head nun or the CEO of the hospital had made that demand but from what I've put together since, and the fact that several of my other long-term partners were booted out not long thereafter, it seemed that a coup d'etat was in the works. And while it came as a shock, and I made an attempt, talking with legal counsel about fighting it, it turned out to be a very positive personal and career move.

On my last day of work, I'd uncharacteristically developed a bad gastroenteritis, with cramping and diarrhea. I say uncharacteristically because for all the years I was working in the ER, exposed to god knows what variety of infectious diseases, I barely ever was sick. I tend to believe that all those exposures boosted my immune system. That day, however, I felt like crap, almost didn't come in. When I showed up my partner Fang took one look at me and said, "Ken, just go into one of the rooms in the back, and I'll take care of everything."

So, there I sat, in an unused part of the large ER, IV in my arm, getting meds and fluids and gradually feeling better. As I lay there, it began to feel like I was in effect "holding court". When the rest of the ER crew heard I was sick, all my fellow workers began coming in whenever they had free time to sit and reminisce with me. I have lovely photos from that night, a lot of smiles and affection, and sadness, from us all, knowing that after that shift I'd be gone.

Right after that, there was a big party thrown for me by the nurses at a local restaurant. My buddies brought in a variety of gifts and mementos. One that I still have is a huge white bed sheet on which everyone from the ER wrote, in multicolored magic marker, their favorite Ken phrases, patient encounters, or other memories. John Poole made sure to be there and gave a truly endearing speech about how, to him, I embodied what the Holy Name ER stood for. The Director, who'd claimed he had no choice but to let me go, showed up uninvited, and we had a very bittersweet interaction.

All in all, the love I felt from the nurses, PAs, and my other colleagues, touched me deeply and made me see how much they valued me as a coworker and more importantly, how much I meant to them.

When this more formal event ended, there was a lovely, looser party at one of the nurses' houses. It went on so late into the night that I wound up crashing in her spare room. I woke up the next morning and drove up the New York State Throughway back to Old Chatham, beginning to sense that being let go after all that time was going to be incredibly liberating.

And while I continued to do ER work for another year or two, in other New York and New Jersey Emergency Departments, initially not wanting to totally walk away from all I'd learned/acquired in those 30 years, it quickly became clear that it was time for the next chapter.

CHAPTER 32

URGENT CARING

After leaving Holy Name, I worked a few more years at other ERs, both in NY and NJ. I was desperate to stop, I was in the midst of a nasty divorce, my daughter had gone off to boarding school, and despite my writing, my piano lessons, frequent bike rides, and time Upstate, at that point, I was feeling out of control, mentally unhealthy and self-indulgent. While going through this, I was also trying to date women I was meeting on Match and other sites and not doing very well in those encounters at all. In fact, I think I could write a whole book called *Mismatch*, documenting the amazing lunacy, deception, and thoughtlessness that occurred in those encounters. One thing that I did learn from this, however, was to *never* date a woman whose father had been a muckety muck in the CIA. I inadvertently dated two!

Luckily, one of my colleagues from one of my last emergency rooms, Palisades General, told me, "Ken, I'm going to get you out of the ER and find you a great woman to be with."

Sure enough, I soon was walking to work at his urgent care a few blocks from where I was living in the West Village, and he introduced me to his older sister.

Neither of his two proposals worked out for long but I quickly and mercifully got involved in the world of urgent care. This was often at locations, for the first time in my career, a walk or subway ride from home. And I was no longer dealing with the overwhelming lunacy of the ER.

Unfortunately, and not surprisingly though, I found that most of the urgent cares, while run by MDs, had their own major issues. While the original intentions may have been to create a setting that provided quick, efficient, and competent care, the profit motive was now the basic driver of everything. There was often not enough staff, terrible or inadequate supplies, and a constant push, push, push to see more patients.

Even CityMD, where I worked for several years, was a mill, run by a cabal of docs at the top, with very little interest in feedback from below. And while I met great MDs there, it soon became clear that the physicians in charge had their own agenda and were only concerned with their brand to ultimately be bought out by a conglomerate. They wanted MDs who'd come in, not take lunch breaks, and see one patient after another for anywhere from 8-14 hours at a time. Not a very healthy environment. All in all, when I count back, I worked for 5 or 6 different urgent care companies (ironically, when I was still at Holy Name, it became clear that urgent cares were going to explode in popularity. My ex-partner, Tony Azar, began one with which I was involved, and then not, and then my ex-friend Mario Miglietta and I started one. Unfortunately, due to my own terrible business acumen, a front desk person who was stealing from us, and a sociopathic associate who helped undermine the whole venture, we opened and closed our own urgent care, Riverfront Medical Associates in Edgewater after about two years).

Luckily, I started working for my friend, Neal Shipley, who ran two urgent care locations in Manhattan. I could walk to work at one of them and even after the urgent care was taken over by Northwell, with all the politics and issues attendant in a large hospital chain, Neal was still around, and I work there still (doing telemedicine).

I read a piece recently that hit the nail on the head about the relationship between medical practitioners and administrators. Most administrators know or quickly learn that the majority of MDs, PAs, NPs, nurses, and techs, are a dedicated bunch. Either they start out like that, or they develop the trait along the way. This gives those administrators a lot of leeway in terms of not feeling the pressure to provide adequate supplies, or techs or other staff. They know that the people working will do pretty much anything to make do, to compensate, to take their own X-rays, draw their own labs, anything to ensure that patients get proper care. It's a dynamic easily abused, as I've seen throughout my career, as it's happened countless times to me and my colleagues. It's one of the worst things about working in medicine, and I don't know that there is anything that will ever change it.

Even having said that, I know I've helped countless patients, mentored many practitioners, and made a lot of people laugh, even under the worst of circumstances. And even though, with my often just below-the-surface Jewish guilt that I should still be doing something more, I generally can accept that moving towards my 77th year to heaven, I, like so many in my profession, keep giving it my all, the pleasure, satisfaction, and gratitude from patients and their families keeps most of us going.

Herewith are some of my stories from the varied world of Urgent Care:

CHAPTER 33

Saturday Storms

One Saturday morning, after I'd been working in the Midwood section of Brooklyn for about 6 months, I heard the news about the deaths of seven Jewish children there, the night before.

I was practicing Urgent Care medicine, after thirty years as an ER physician, and now found myself, a secular Jew, surrounded by my more observant brethren: Hasids, Orthodox, both traditional and Modern, Conservatives and Reform.

An interloper from Manhattan, on Saturday mornings I'd drive down Ocean Parkway and Coney Island Avenue past streets filled with men in beaver hats and long coats as they walked to shul. It would feel like my trip across the East River hadn't taken me to another borough, but to another world, one in which I'd find myself curious, bemused, often uncomprehending, and after the deadly fire, horrified.

It seemed that an unquestioning adherence to the *Shulchan Aruch* (literally the "set table" or legal codes derived from the written and oral Torah that Orthodox Jews use to govern their daily lives) had caused otherwise intelligent, rational, well-meaning people to behave in ways ruled by magical thinking.

That Friday night, the behavior ended in disastrous results. A hotplate left on in the kitchen (to avoid using an electrical switch on Shabbos), had burst into flames after the family had gone to bed, and the ensuing conflagration had killed the children sleeping upstairs.

Over the time I'd been working in Brooklyn, I came to accept the fact that the bagel store isn't open Friday morning or that the Dunkin Donuts on Kings Highway won't serve any meat. I learned that the sign in the tailor's window advertising Shadnez testing means that customers may bring their garments in, sale tags still on, to see if there is any linen thread used to sew together the woolen suits. This is a practice forbidden by the Shulchan Aruch. If that taboo mix is discovered the clothes must be returned to the store unworn. And I was told about the three Eruvs in Brooklyn. These are lines strung up on telephone poles to demarcate areas where religious Jews can avoid the proscription against carrying anything, be it babies, parcels, or prayer books, on Shabbos, practices they'd otherwise have to avoid.

Interestingly, after a storm in New Jersey's Bergen County caused the local Eruv there to fall to the ground, I read a piece in *The New York Times* about the Orthodox mothers who were having a Talmudic debate about whether they could behave as if the line was still up.

The Saturday following the Friday night fire, I had a patient who was very upset, and needing my guidance. She wanted to be sure that she hadn't done anything wrong by coming in on Shabbos with part of a Q-tip stuck in her ear. I tried in my Non-observant Jewish way to reassure her but to no avail. It was only when I informed her that, by my flushing the material out of her ear canal, preventing a potential infection, that she was truly relieved. She left that day feeling that she had not gone against any of the commandments, by her visit to me in urgent care.

All of these interactions and other surrounding events in the religious community have caused a mix of feelings and thoughts: I have been outraged at the Orthodox Jews' apparent complicity with child molesters within their midst; have been horrified by the unwillingness of fellow Jews to name the moyls (men trained to do ritual circumcision) responsible for the deaths of the Jewish infants from herpes transmitted to them through an ancient and dubious practice of sucking the blood from the circumcised penis of newborns during the bris, by these moyls. On the other hand, I was surprised and delighted one day by my interaction with one of my patients. He was an elderly Orthodox man, a professor and yet, during a conversation about literature we began, he shared with me a love of Jean Genet, the very unorthodox French author. Plus, at the Midwood facility, I worked with tremendously dedicated and experienced Modern Orthodox Physician Assistants, women whom I'd come to admire as they bridged the gap between the solemn tenets of Judaism and their equally compelling needs and desires to have meaningful, fulfilling careers in medicine.

After I'd watched the news of the fire that day, I was having trouble not seeing the seven children's deaths as the result of archaic beliefs, something caused by behavior rooted in superstition and a refusal to adapt to modern times. The ultimate and most exalted conduct an Orthodox Jew can engage in is to spend the entirety of one's life reading the scriptures to truly understand them, yet it's acknowledged that very few can achieve this goal. If that is so then, for those who cannot attain that deepest understanding, isn't all of life a compromise, a slippery slope? Having lost the battle to be the most truly pious, obedient Jew, how does one pick and choose which tenets to continue to obey? And if choice is involved in the goal to be as pious as possible, how can lives be lost over a hotplate?

All of this swirled around in my mind that Saturday, as more details about the deaths were filtering in. When my shift ended that evening, I headed back towards Manhattan and drove down a Coney Island Avenue that now, with Shabbos over, was alive and festive, streets filled with Jewish men and women of all ages happily hurrying home. I began to wonder if the seven children's demise was the predictable result of behavior based on obsolete and archaic, religious thinking or, like the following week's events (the horrific deaths of 150 people in the French Alps plane crash, the nightmare of the buildings blowing up in the East Village from a gas main and the two deaths there) were just one of those random occurrences that bring tragedy down on any of us, religious or not, as we merely try to lead our rational, humane, daily lives.

CHAPTER 34

What The Right Hand Doesn't Know

It was a hot, humid summer Saturday in the Upper West Side Urgent Care. By mid-afternoon, it was clear that few patients would be braving the heat to see us.

I was sitting in the back of the facility, drinking an iced coffee and kibitzing with my colleagues when the sensor by the front door pinged, alerting us of a possible patient arrival.

A few minutes later, Jamal, who'd been manning the reception desk, walked over to me.

"Doctor Weinberg, I have a religious Jewish family here. Father's a doctor. Their son has a nasty sore throat, and they want to register him as a patient."

"We're happy to see him. Is there an issue?" I asked.

"The problem is that because it's the Sabbath the dad says he can't sign the HIPPA form."

"He's gotta sign it," I responded. "That's the policy. And my understanding is that in Jewish law illness trumps any religious restrictions, so there's no reason that he can't do it if he wants his son to be evaluated."

With that information in hand, Jamal retraced his steps.

I sat, mulling over the situation, curious to hear what was next.

"Okay, Doc," Jamal allowed as he returned. "The father says he can sign. He'll just do it with his left hand."

'Holy shit!' I thought, 'What a brilliant way for him to circumvent the Shabbos dilemma.'

My colleagues were equally impressed by this bit of legerdemain, and as I waited for the family to be put into a room and triaged, I told them about another Shabbos conundrum I'd been privy to. It had occurred a few years earlier when I was working at a different Urgent Care, also on Manhattan's Upper West Side.

That day I'd had a patient who was a middle-aged, yarmulked attorney. When I walked into his treatment room, I noticed that he was reading the Op-ed section in *The New York Times*, a provocative combination in my mind. As we spoke about what had brought him in, I became intrigued by what I felt were the many disparate seeming facets of his persona (his own ability to hold on to a paradox). He was liberal, up on current events but was religiously observant and lived with his mother. It wasn't busy that day, so after examining him I started up a conversation about Jewish law, and my sense that it seemed to proscribe or prohibit one's ability to address pressing health issues on the Sabbath.

At this comment, he smiled and plunged into a story about the specific prohibition regarding schmearing on Shabbos: "I had a bad infection on the behind a few years ago. Had to put an antibiotic ointment on the skin back there three times a day. It was fine to do this six days a week but once sundown approached on Friday, I wasn't allowed to directly place anything medicinal on my body for 24 hours. No schmearing."

"What did you do?" I asked, immediately conjuring up an image of the potential ravages caused by an inadequately treated infection on the tuchas. Up till then, all I knew from schmearing was putting cream cheese on a bagel.

"Did you figure out a way around it?"

"Actually, I did," he replied.

"Just before dark on Friday I'd go into the bathroom, take the antibiotic ointment, and squeeze out a dollop on some wax paper. I'd lay that paper on the closed toilet seat. Then, I'd take my pants down a bit and sit on the ointment-covered paper."

I was struck by his ingenuity. But the ingenuity felt to me like it was motivated by a large dose of magical thinking (does God really care if you schmear the paper or schmear your behind?)

Then with an ironic grin, he'd said in summation:

"That's why there are so many Jewish attorneys. We are constantly debating and interpreting Talmudic law."

As I drew back from this memory I thought:

‘Of course! If the lawyer could do that with the schmear, it wouldn’t be much more of a reach for the father to switch signature hands so he could have his child seen today on Shabbos.’

And I realized, ‘What a great example of the right hand not knowing what the left hand is doing!’

I didn’t anticipate what would happen next that afternoon, however.

I entered my new patient’s room and after brief introductions took a look in his throat. Jamal had already done a swab and when I turned to check the results, I saw it had turned conclusively positive for strep. Turning back, I told the anxious parents that their son’s nasty, pus-covered tonsils needed immediate antibiotic treatment.

The father smiled as if he’d known that all along, then (clearly sensing what our response would be) he looked first at his wife, then at me, and asked:

“Well...Doctor Weinberg, do you think we can afford to wait until after Shabbos sundown tonight to give him the first dose of Cefdinir?”

I don’t recall if the wife shouted “No!” first or I did but based on our mutual response I feel certain that as soon as they left the urgent care, they immediately headed across the street to the nearest pharmacy to get in that first dose stat!

CHAPTER 35

Erectile Tissue

One early Spring, I was working in my fourth or fifth Urgent Care practice. I'd moved to the Upper West Side, where I could still walk to work, but I found myself doing things that, had I still been in the ER, I would have considered beneath me, things I would have expected a nurse or even an orderly, to do.

This day was particularly busy, and I was taking a much-needed break when I saw a new patient arrive. As he came through the front doors, I couldn't help noticing him: a pleasant-looking, elderly man, with glasses and thick white hair, moving adroitly on a motorized cart. I watched as he began navigating the turns leading to the back examination rooms, accompanied by his wife who was walking briskly just behind him.

As soon as he was triaged, I followed after them, entered his room, and found them at some distance from one another. She was standing in the far corner and her husband sat on his device, now tightly wedged between the sink and the large examining table in the middle of the room.

As I placed myself in another corner, he introduced himself and did most of the talking.

"Nice to meet you, Dr. Weinberg. Just so you know, I have Multiple Sclerosis," he began. "Have had it since 1959. In fact, I just recently visited one of the local medical schools so the students could see that there were actually some patients with MS who could lead long and productive lives, despite the well-known ravages of the disease."

He continued, "Unfortunately, as you also know, there are many unforeseen consequences of MS, and I now have one of them."

As he spoke, I observed he had a metal brace attached to a strap on his right leg which extended to a bulky, thick-soled black shoe. He pointed to the shoe and said that recently, the chafing of his heel from the shoe had started causing him pain. His son, a thoracic surgeon, who'd been visiting from out of town, had done an initial evaluation, felt it was a minor wound, and recommended that he put moleskin on it.

The patient had followed his advice, but the pain had been steadily increasing and the son, no longer around, had told his father that he needed to have another medical evaluation.

I quickly realized that the only way I could see the affected heel would be to kneel on the floor to give a look. As I got on my hands and knees, I also learned that the man was incapable of removing the orthopedic device himself. Glancing over at his wife, I saw that she was staring off into space, clearly not interested in helping. I was flummoxed, afraid to cause more problems if I wrenched the shoe off incorrectly and suddenly wished that I was back in the ER where all of this probably would have been done by an aide or a nurse, the foot exposed for my evaluation even before I entered the room. Urgent Cares generally can't provide this luxury, however.

Fortunately, at his suggestion, and still on my knees tightly tucked between his motorized device and the sink, I was able to leverage the metal rod against the oversized shoe to unearth his foot. I then gently removed the compression stocking beneath it to finally see the heel.

As an ER doc I always expect the worst. I was sure I'd find a gaping wound, reddened and draining pus, but instead was delightfully surprised to find a small, well-healing abrasion.

We continued our conversation, both of us thrilled that no major intervention was needed. He told me that he'd recently retired as a professor at an Upstate medical school.

"What did you teach?" I inquired.

"Physiology," was his reply.

"About neurological illness?' I asked, thinking that his MS might have spurred him to investigate and possibly look for treatments for the disease he had.

"Not really. My field was the olfactory nerve," he responded.

"Interesting," I said. "I was always intrigued that it was the only one of the sensory nerves in the head that went directly into the brain, that there was no synapse between nose and brain and that caused olfactory memories to be so powerful. No modulation before they hit the olfactory cortex in our brain..."

As we talked, I remembered a smell that I could still bring up of the linoleum covering the back staircase of my childhood home in Newark in the '50s. Though we'd moved when I was five (long over sixty years before) anytime the image of that back stairway leading up to the mysterious apartment above us passed through my brain, it always provoked the smell of the linoleum.

"Yeah, my sense of smell is nearly gone," he told me. "Seems to fade with age..."

As I began to clean the wound and apply bacitracin, I told him how, after reading a piece by the writer and physician Lewis Thomas in his book Lives of a Cell, I'd learned that there was erectile tissue in the nose. It had become a source of amusement to me and several friends since this discovery, leading to jokes about nasal stuffiness and sneezing in many inopportune moments.

As I recounted this to him, he replied, "You know, especially at night, the arousal in the erectile tissue seems to migrate from nostril to nostril."

Temporarily shifting my attention from his foot, I looked at him and asked what he meant. "Did you ever notice, during the night, how one nostril gets stuffed for about 20 minutes and then the other?"

I was still on the floor as this discussion was going on and at this point, I had begun the delicate job of pulling his stocking back over the heel, trying desperately not to dislodge my bandaged ministrations. My patient continued explaining the role of erectile tissue in the nose and I suddenly had another realization.

My initial reaction to doing all of this was how demeaning being on the floor was, something (literally) below me, something a scribe or medical assistant (or the patient's wife?) should do. The doctor should not be lowering himself to the floor to do this. Not only would I have never done it in the crazy, well-staffed emergency rooms I'd worked in, but even now it felt like something I had neither the time nor the role to play, on a busy day in Urgent Care.

Yet, here I was literally at his feet, the feet of the Olfactory Nerve Master, learning about erectile tissue in the nose. Levering his bulky shoe back up onto his foot once more so as not to disturb the wound, I had an image of Jesus, washing the feet of lepers. It suddenly became a transformative, reflective, and deeply satisfying moment. It caused me, in ways I'd never considered during my thirty-five years as a physician, to reassess my role in a most humbling, yet gratifying way.

It reminded me of a conversation I'd had several years before with my youngest brother Marc, now deceased. Marc was, before his death, an astonishingly well-respected and beloved family practitioner and healer. At the time of our conversation, we were celebrating the wedding of his daughter. She had just graduated from medical school and

Marc, and his wife were throwing a four-day extravaganza at their home in Sarasota. His daughter (who had just become the fourth generation of Drs. Weinberg), was in the back seat of the family car with three of her medical school buddies. Marc and I, sitting up front, were discussing our thoughts on being physicians, long into our careers. I was complaining about the ER and its nearly non-stop chaos, how in the middle of that I too often felt that patients weren't really seeking a doctor, they were demanding a priest. I said how much I disliked finding myself in that position.

At that, Marc had turned to me.

"Kenny, that's what I love about being a doctor the most," he'd said.

Kneeling on the floor of the urgent care that day, his words rushed back, and I understood once again my brother's wisdom and humility.

CHAPTER 36

Schmeckle Down

It was the week of the High Holy Days.

Not being an observant Jew, I found myself working both the Rosh Hashanah and now, Yom Kippur, shifts in the Urgent Care where I'd been employed for several years.

The day was unfolding in a most unrighteous manner. Unlike a religiously ordained "Day of Atonement," spent among fellow congregants, with services led by a rabbi, where I could ruminate on, and try to expiate my sins, it had become instead a day of personal atonement, and regret, for my showing up to work at all on a Jewish holiday.

I was the only physician at the site, and I had only one assistant to help deal with the overwhelming number of incoming patients. Plus, we'd walked in to find there were inadequate medical supplies and no radiology technician to take any needed X-rays.

Adding to my regret was the realization early in the shift that, despite multiple phone calls, emails, and texts from me to the Powers That Be about our dire and dangerous situation, no help would be forthcoming. I was feeling a deep sense of abandonment, of being thrown to the wolves on this holiest of days.

"What a fool I was to decide to labor on Yom Kippur," I mused. "Perhaps someone is trying to tell me something."

Though I strongly self-identify as Jewish, I long ago realized the rituals in shul during the High Holy Days—rituals that for many are a reflective, cleansing experience—only leave me flat. When I'd submitted my schedule requests the prior month, I hadn't given a thought about working on Rosh Hashanah or Yom Kippur and hadn't even realized what dates they were.

As the nightmare of the day, tolling on The Yom (as some people call it) unfolded, I was kicking myself, becoming more and more angered. Prescriptions weren't going through to the pharmacies, patients were sicker, nastier, and more demanding than usual.

I realized I was at least partly to blame though, as I'd foolishly assumed when I walked in to start the twelve-hour shift that day, it would be relatively slow. I'd expected that the largely Jewish population on the Upper West Side of Manhattan (where the urgent care is located) would be more focused on synagogue than sickness. Instead, we were exceptionally busy, and nearly out of control.

By 7:00 p.m., I was raw, drained, and having problems being my usual caring, even jovial self. I was desperate for the shift to end. Fortunately, there was a lull at that moment, and I walked to the back of the facility, in hopes of catching up on my charting so I could bolt out the door on time at 8:00.

I was sitting in front of my computer, clicking nimbly as I signed off on my charts when I became aware of a new patient registering at the front desk. As I listened to the sound of his voice and heard what I sensed was the self-induced desperation of his circumstances, I was primed for aggravation when I walked in to see him.

I trudged into the room and found him sitting casually on the examining table. His tattered shirt was partly open to reveal a mass of mangled, soiled tape and gauze dressings, hanging off the left side of his chest and abdomen. He was a wizened, scruffy, little bald-haired man, of indeterminate age—though from his chart I quickly discovered he was in his mid-sixties.

He told me he was half Irish Catholic, half Jewish, and lived deep in Brooklyn. As I stepped closer to him, he began revealing his story, explaining why he had felt forced to come all the way to our urgent care, and informing me about his recent surgery to remove a testicular tumor. He bemoaned the episodic, inadequate treatment he'd had since the procedure due to his being on Medicaid, and his recent inability to get the right supplies to cover the wounds he'd incurred after a complicated operation gone wrong.

His saga and the obvious inequities he'd suffered only added to my annoyance and frustration, an annoyance that was growing (and showing) as he disrobed entirely to reveal a surgical scar that extended from scrotum to nipple, taking up much of the left side of his groin and abdomen. At that point, I began to get an actual sense of what he'd been going through, and I also realized that properly caring for that wound was going to take me way past our 8 PM official closing time.

Always the professional though, I began formulating a plan for what had to be done. And as I pondered the situation, I found that in spite of myself, I was starting to warm to him.

He watched me as I inspected his extensive cicatrix, and as I turned towards a cabinet to get the supplies I'd need, he asked:

"How does it look, doc?"

"It could be a lot worse," I allowed.

"Have you read any Shakespeare? *Romeo and Juliet*?"

"Yes," I said, though I couldn't at that moment recall when.

"Do you remember the dialogue between Mercutio and Romeo after Mercutio's been stabbed?"

I had to admit I didn't.

So, he proceeded to recite it to me. Verbatim, with a near-perfect-pitch English accent.

Romeo: Courage, man; the hurt cannot be much.

Mercutio: No, 'tis not so deep as a well, nor so wide as a church door; but 'tis enough, 'twill serve. Ask for me tomorrow, and you shall find me a grave man.

With that he had me. At that moment he could have asked me for anything, and it would have been his. I hunkered down, assiduously cleaning the dirt from his wound, and then, even though we had none of the large, yellow gauze dressings he needed, I began covering in a most patchwork quilt manner, his reddened, raw scar, from a deformed scrotum, past a contorted umbilicus and up to a mangled left nipple, with our own tiny, oily pads. As I toiled, he soliloquized about his gigs as a standup comic, about his unorthodox religious and cultural upbringing, about his maniacal hatred for Trump...

Ironically, listening to him talk as I performed one of the things most proscribed on this holiest of days, washing him, and feeling us bond while I scrupulously cared for the wounds, it was as if I was being given the chance to wash away my own transgressions from the past year.

At one point, far into these ministrations, I had to lift up his post-surgical penis to clean what was left of the scrotum, then cover it with gauze. I needed his assistance when I completed that task.

"Schmeckle down," I requested.

He complied and rearranging himself, his remaining testicle, and his schmeckle, he began riffing on what the down from a schmeckle (compared to say, goose down) would be like. I'm not sure I can repeat, nor would care to, the imagery he evoked as I continued the process of covering and then taping down his dressings. I will say though, that by the time I was done, having placed countless lubricated gauze squares over the left side of his groin and torso, covered them with dry dressings, and then secured them in place with yards and yards of tape, I found myself transformed. I vowed to go home, and reread Romeo and Juliet and I left work that night feeling refreshed, uplifted, and absolved.

As I walked home, I realized it was my own perfect Yom Kippur.

CHAPTER 37

THE CLEARNESS COMMITTEE

I found another way, besides writing, to keep my sanity as my time in the ER was coming to an end. This is through my ongoing involvement in a group called Courage to Lead (CTL).

CTL was started in the 90s by Penny Williamson, who had a doctorate in Biology and Ecology from Johns Hopkins and was working with medical communities (especially the American Board of Internal Medicine). trying to enhance the medical paradigm. She was introduced to, and taken by, the power of a nearly 400-year-old Quaker practice known as The Clearness Committee. She saw how the Committee could open up participants to much deeper levels of understanding, helping them to resolve particularly thorny issues. It became clear to Penny that retreats incorporating the Clearness Committee could be truly beneficial to the people in the medical community she'd been working with.

Soon she was joined by Dr. Hanna Sherman. Hanna had been working, both in the United States and internationally, on ways to create safe spaces for personal and professional growth and develop personal and collective wisdom in the healthcare community. Her vision was complementary to Penny's, and they began leading these interactive retreats together.

CTL consists of a series of gatherings that originally took place over eighteen months on Cape Cod. Each one was open to twelve participants and was held at a lovely 1848 Victorian B&B in Sandwich, close to the national seashore. The sessions would explore how one's inner life and outer work connect; ways to find joy and fulfillment in leadership roles and activities; and how to bring one's optimal gifts and skills to bear at work in a way that not only sustains courage but allows all those capacities to be modeled for others (both colleagues and mentees). In addition, taking advantage of the fact that the retreats occurred during Fall, Winter, Spring, and Summer, they would integrate themes that look at the deeper meanings and associations that each of the four seasons represents.

What makes CTL special is its central tenet: the use of the Clearness Committee, the concept evolved by the Quaker community so many years ago in New England. The Committee, consisting of three to seven members, would be called together whenever someone within the community had an issue they couldn't resolve themselves and needed objective, but heartfelt, guidance on. Once a Committee was set in motion there was a standardized pattern to how things would proceed: After a period of quiet reflection, or centering silence in the group, the person who'd requested the Committee would lay out his or her problem. The members would listen as the issue was fully articulated and then ask questions. These were never questions the members themselves thought they knew the answer to. Instead, they would be open-ended, honest (and often not rational, but intuitive) questions, designed to get the person to reflect on the matter from a different angle. In addition, and critical to its unique ability to bring insight to the member, the group would meet within a framework of "double confidentiality." This meant that, after the session ended no one would discuss any of it within the group or outside and would only re-engage about it if the subject of the Clearness Committee brought it up to one of the participating members.

Hanna and Penny had been leading these interactive retreats together for about 15 years when, sometime in the Summer of 2011, my friend Sara W. told me about them. Sara had just completed the year and 1/2 retreat, had found it very meaningful, and thought I might find it to be as well.

On Sara's recommendation, I looked at the curriculum and the roster of people who'd attended in the past. They were leaders in academic medicine and allied fields, people with very impressive resumes. I wasn't sure I'd make the grade, might not have enough to bring to the group. But I applied anyway, including my *New York Times* article on my father's death to show some kind of bona fides, and to my surprise, was accepted.

This was at a time when I was feeling very isolated. I had just been fired, after twenty-two years, from Holy Name Hospital. I was working at other ERs, living more Upstate than in Manhattan, was grappling with my self-worth and worth as a physician. I had increasingly been feeling I was being called upon more as a priest than an MD, feeling like my soul was being sucked out, as I felt more and more put upon by the inhumane medical structures within which I worked.

I felt that my patients and their families, especially those dealing with chronic medical issues, were being hurt, and crushed, not just medically but spiritually, and when they showed up in the ER my role needed to be not just trying to fix or help their acute medical problems but the deep psychic pain they were in as well.

And while at times I was aware of a sense (that had imperceptibly seeped into my being over the years), that I had so much to bring to the table as a doc, I also, especially after being fired unceremoniously, felt that I wasn't appreciated, nor was I getting paid anyway near what I deserved at that point in my career. In short, I was feeling my self-love and self-respect being shredded.

I began CTL amid those events and feelings that Fall and thus began, what should have been a year and a half immersive journey, but for a core group of us continues to this day, fifteen years later. After the Cape Cod location was no longer available, we did a retreat in Aspen, then several years in Old Chatham, and now this Spring will have our second get-together in the Smokie Mountains in North Carolina.

At the start of the initial three-day retreats, we'd get together over breakfast, then break into a circle of twelve, talking about touchstones that we have come to understand were critical to our health-related practices, and our lives. Penny and Hannah would weave certain themes into the sessions. These were taken from the work of Parker Palmer (who first introduced Penny and Hanna to the Clearance Committee) or using the writing of Alice Walker, Rilke, Rumi, poets Billy Collins, Mary Oliver, Robert Frost ("two roads diverged in a yellow wood") or one time, a video showing the work of artist Andy Goldsboro. We'd write to prompts based on these themes and sometimes color in our journals, reflect on the readings, and then discuss them. We'd break for lunch, go for walks along the beautiful Cape Cod coastline, and explore the Town of Sandwich. We'd look for transformative objects on the beach, reflect on what we'd been discussing that day, meet again in the afternoon, and enjoy the great food and drink that was served three times a day at The Isaiah Jones House. At night we'd schmooze, play music, and get to know one another. After my hip surgery, when I was no longer limping along as I had been on the prior retreat, we all celebrated by indulging in a long group dance to some great old rock and roll.

Despite our different backgrounds, ages, and geographic locations (West Coast, Midwest, Canada, the South) and points of view (though it quickly became clear that we all felt most allied with progressive and humanistic approaches to the world,) over the course of the retreats we became extremely close, respectful, and fond of one another.

Of course, working this closely together brought up some profound personal material and the group would be encouraged to reflect on it in ways we'd never considered before. One memorable example was the concept of holding on to a paradox. We were prompted to think of and write about an occasion when this had occurred in our lives. As is frequently the case with these prompts, I had to think hard and reach back in my memory to find a situation where this had happened to me. And then it hit me. I remembered an event several years earlier that highlighted my ability to balance two opposing ideas and how fragile that balance could be:

On the last Sunday in August of 2006, I had flown down to Florida to see my father, who was approaching the end of his life. I was sitting with him in his bedroom in Delray Beach, a setting I'd been in countless times since they'd moved from South Orange probably twenty years earlier. The day before I arrived my father had, in disgust, left the hospital where he'd been admitted a few days earlier to control his increasingly frequent intestinal bleeding. He'd left because he felt that nothing was being done for him. On that Saturday night, he'd asked my brother Neil to bring him some (forbidden) beer and pizza. Neil surreptitiously brought it into his hospital room and Neil, my mother, and my father consumed it. Immediately after this, my father took off his hospital gown, ripped off his name band, and unceremoniously signed himself out against medical advice.

It was now Sunday afternoon, and he and I were talking casually, kibitzing as we often did about medicine, family, or politics. I was having this conversation, looking out the window at our ping pong table, the pool and palms and fruit trees beyond it, as if nothing would ever change. It would be South Florida, my mother, brothers, their wives and kids all hanging out, eating ridiculously sumptuous meals at the clubhouse, going to the beach and body surfing, eating my mother's amazing signature ice cream cake.

We were acting as if all was fine, and yet, somewhere in the back of my mind, I knew my father was dying. But on the other hand, he seemed totally intact. And while I regret that I didn't ask him more things about his earlier life (like his experiences as a flight surgeon during World War II) the fact that we could have been sitting there, just talking as father and son, having grown to really respect and appreciate each other after so many years of conflict, felt very special.

Knowing that it would be the last time we might ever do this, meant a tremendous amount to me. We were sitting like we always had, chatting that is, until the moment when the dam burst.

He'd just gotten a phone call from the hematologist's office, and he was upset because they were hocking him to come into the office again, for one more blood draw, maybe another platelet transfusion.

He slammed the phone down and eyed me, frustrated, and angry. "What do they want from me? I'm tired of this crap, don't feel like schlepping over to that fucking office again!"

I looked at him, somewhat surprised by his vociferous response, and replied, "Dad, it's up to you. It's your decision. If you don't want to do this anymore, you don't have to."

When I said that the paradox shattered and exploded in my brain. I was struck by the fact that, though we'd been sitting and talking in his bedroom, this was different. He was dying and I could no longer deny it. At that moment I confronted how the sands were shifting rapidly under our feet, and I lost control and burst into tears.

My father immediately grabbed my shoulder. "Don't cry," he implored me.

I had to stand up and quickly leave the bedroom. I was now sobbing uncontrollably, my whole body shaking as I tramped out into their living room.

I paced for fifteen minutes, wrenching out all of the sadness I could, and then, calm once more, went back into the bedroom and continued the conversation. He died two days later.

Until that day in CTL, I'd never considered the concept (though I see it so often now) of how we all, usually unconsciously, walk around holding on to two seemingly conflicting concepts, more often than I'd ever imagined. And that prompt and discussion of paradox in the group brought it home powerfully.

On the third day of each retreat, we'd convene The Clearness Committee. Whether I was the subject or a member of the group, the concept of being held by my colleagues like you'd hold a fallen baby bird in your hands, eventually allowing it to take flight within the increasingly trusting community we formed, became transformative.

The magic in the Committee is its ability, through open-ended questions, to get someone to be able to truly articulate the truth that they are seeking in a difficult situation. It allows them to uncover their personal "Snowden secret" (if I may borrow that concept from Catch-22) by not just asking those questions but also by the group's use of "mirroring", relaying to the subject what their facial expressions were, or body language expressed, amid the questions and answers. The entire process, including learning the ability to not betray your own prejudices in the questions, not even unconsciously pushing the subject into saying what you want them to say or have felt, has had a lot to do with my own evolving processes in my interactions with patients, my colleagues, and especially the Physician Assistants and Nurse Practitioners who come to me for guidance.

The first time the group met in Old Chatham, in 2016, Georgia and two of her closest friends were nearby and showed up as we were on a break. That was especially meaningful because she finally was able to get a sense of what I'd been doing, and with whom I'd been meeting for all of those years. And what was striking then, as well, was how that coincided with watching my CTL buddies as they took in my house and the 12+ acres surrounding it. My thoughtful, honest friends, walking around, taking in the feeling of the location, reflecting on what a special place I have, and somehow seeing me in a newer, deeper way. Their spoken observations of me, the place, seeing it all through their eyes surprised me. I hadn't thought about how people might react to where I've been living, on or off for over twenty years when I suggested we hold our retreat in Old Chatham. And I was struck by what everyone said, the idea of who I am, my connection to, and what I've done with my house, with its views of forty miles of the Upper Hudson Valley. Those reflections were so generous and unexpectedly delightful.

As I sit writing this, I think about the people who've attended CTL with me, most of them MDs, leaders in their fields, chairs of departments, and others involved in health care policy on a global basis, and I reflect on our ongoing willingness after fifteen years to continue to share so much of our lives and work. And as I look at the writing I did when we began, and the journals I've been keeping for fifty years, I am struck by the effect CTL has had on me and why I keep participating in the retreats. Reading my journals, I can truly see a progression from the start of our retreats, where I was still tense, mostly living in the city, and the angst I was feeling toward the end of my ER career. I could see and feel from the words I wrote then how tranquil I'd be during our retreats. Those fleeting feelings of equilibrium and peace then, even as I was transitioning into Urgent Care and now Medical Cannabis, are no longer so fleeting.

These days I feel secure in my place in Old Chatham and myself, much more centered, grounded, and fulfilled. I've truly come to love the quiet, the stillness, the light, and the views, how they change through the seasons, the large seasonal trajectory the sunsets take, as they set deep and long towards the North in Summer and short and fast so far to the South in Winter. I realize that mostly being here and not so much in the city, allows me to be in touch with my own rhythms, probably for the first time in my life.

And while I still harbor a deep suspicion of how much any person can change, about how much any process can lead to insight, I am astonished, at how much I have actually changed, in my self-confidence, self-love, and humility. That may be the most important change of all, and CTL and its groups were a major part of that transformation.

Each year we are reassured by the knowledge that we will continue to meet and stay open and probing and contemplative with each other into the future and that we'll always have a Clearance Committee where we can hold each one of us like a baby bird.

CHAPTER 38

The Pleasures and Perils of Telemedicine

During the COVID-19 pandemic, I wound up precipitously moving from seeing patients in person in the urgent care setting to only doing telemedicine.

At its onset, in March of 2020, I was working in an Urgent Care on the Upper West Side of Manhattan. The first Friday of that month, there'd been one of the first superspreader events in New York at a Shabbos gathering in New Rochelle.

As I sat in the Urgent Care that Wednesday afternoon, a patient came in. I approached him and asked why he was there.

"You heard about that event in New Rochelle last Friday? I was there."

We had no masks, no gowns, no way of testing for COVID, let alone treating it.

When I told Susan and Georgia about this, they both freaked out. Told me I clearly should not be seeing patients in person any longer. At the age of 70, having recently had both the base of my aorta and aortic valve replaced, I was clearly at high risk and needed to abandon the direct patient care setting I'd worked in for thirty-five years.

Susan also said, "Oh, and while you're at it, I think you should flee the city as well. Go and live in the house in Old Chatham."

I was happy to take her advice. I love Old Chatham, and it was the start of Spring there, my favorite season. Also, as luck would have it, with the incredible, nearly immediate stress COVID put on the country's healthcare system, the Federal Government very quickly made it much easier to use a variety of platforms for telemedicine. As was hoped for, telemedicine would prove to be a great complement and reliever of pressure for the nation's now overwhelmed healthcare facilities and providers.

While 5-10 minute online patient interactions have yet to lend themselves to full-blown stories, I have had very meaningful encounters, clinically and emotionally gratifying:

One afternoon, I saw a patient online with right ear pain. As he and I discussed, I obviously could not see his ears or throat. But his voice sounded muffled to me, and I was concerned he could have an abscess on his right tonsil. I told him he needed to be seen in person and was informed later that day that he in fact had a large abscess on his right tonsil that was immediately opened and drained.

Experiences like that make me feel good about my 40 years of medical experience and how, even without being able to lay my hands on someone, my diagnostic acumen seems to remain sharp.

On the second Christmas Eve of the year after the pandemic hit, we were in a rebound from 2 years of COVID isolation. By this point, COVID, Flu, and RSV were wreaking havoc on the entire system. I'd been reading that there was no amoxicillin, Tamiflu or Motrin in pharmacies. Everyone was sick as hell, the ERs were overcrowded, Urgent Cares overflowing, and telemedicine was again providing an escape valve for the system.

That night, I had just gotten off a call with a patient, a 26-year-old woman with a totally obscure autoimmune disease, one I'd never heard of before. This woman, who lived alone, had developed a fever the night before, took a gram of Tylenol, and despite that, had a seizure. She'd initiated this virtual visit because she still had a fever. And while she'd worked as an EMT, was obviously very smart, and knew her disease well, she wanted advice. It was clear to me that she needed to go to the ER, but she seemed to need to hear it directly and explicitly. I reminded her of all the potential risks she was running and gently told her she had to go. She assured me she would, and I signed off the call, glad to know she'd take my advice.

That encounter was immediately followed by what turned out to be my second visit with a patient who I'd first seen six days prior. The first time had occurred late in the afternoon on the day his elderly father had suddenly died, at home, in front of him. When I had reached him online on the day of visit #1, I learned, in between the coughing fits I was watching and hearing, that he had only made this appointment with me at his wife's insistence. His cough had been getting worse, and they were thinking that steroids would help. As we spoke, I thought about how he must be feeling, having this persistent, worsening cough that he was trying to minimize, a father whom he'd just seen die that morning, and a mother and brother he was trying to comfort. My heart went out to him. I was very concerned about what could be causing the cough.

As we now met again on the screen for visit #2, he told me that since I'd initially seen him, despite his having been put on steroids, the cough had worsened. I also discovered that since I'd last seen him, he'd buried his father, and that, unsurprisingly, his mother and brother, and he, were still in shock from the death but were attempting to move on.

This scenario was all relayed to me against a backdrop of his frequent paroxysms of cough, still unrelieved by prednisone.

"Doc, can you just give me more steroids for a few days, please?"

I told him, "The worst thing about telemedicine, and I say this as an ER doc for over 30 years, is that I can't examine you, don't have a good explanation for your persistent symptoms, and can't rule out pneumonia or any other serious processes that could be going on. Giving you steroids might only make things worse."

I also expressed my concern once more for the overwhelming amount of stress he was going through. With that comment, he began to cry. I watched, in surprise, as he took a Kleenex to his eyes.

I'd clearly triggered something.

"Doctor, thank you for what you are saying. Your caring is really touching. You know you are part of a dying breed."

I know that he said much more, but my own emotions got carried away at that moment as well, and I can't recall what else he told me.

I thanked him, deeply, paused, and then said,

"OK. But now you really need to go be seen. How soon can you get to Urgent Care? I'll contact them immediately and make sure all is taken care of."

Shortly thereafter, my patient went in, was examined, and received his needed chest X-ray. The exam and X-ray were fortunately normal. Now we had a justification for his getting more steroids. I was relieved to know that he had finally been taken care of, in time to go home for his muted, I am sure, Christmas Eve dinner.

Apart from this type of unusually emotional encounter in the online world, there is another strange phenomenon I first noticed in the urgent care that persists online.

Patients or family members will appear in front of me on the screen who are clearly very ill and in need of immediate in-person interventions. They have chest pain, difficulty breathing, or have just developed weakness in an arm or leg, and yet they have made appointments to be seen virtually. They want me to tell them that any of those symptoms don't mean anything, not heart attack, pulmonary embolism, or stroke. They are in a fine, acutely developed state of denial, and they want me to authenticate it. They want me to tell them it's okay, that they don't really need to call the ambulance.

I couldn't initially understand this when I was first confronted it online but quickly realized that this was analogous to what I'd seen in person in the urgent care: patients who had to know they were sick, with symptoms that on some level they sensed were really serious, but still, they would show up in the clinic despite this.

I came to realize that they were looking for a pass. It's an amazing phenomenon, not uncommon. And I am no longer shocked or horrified when I realize they are doing it. I've come to realize they were hoping, denial being such a strong motivator, that I would give them that pass, and validate their denial.

I've come to realize that they wanted so badly not to admit, or acknowledge the deadly implications of their symptoms, that they decided to see a practitioner, not in the emergency room where down deep they knew they belonged, but instead in a setting that implied much less, or no acuity, of the severity of symptoms. They'd come to us in the belief that we could allay their fears and tell them it was nothing serious, and they could just go home. It was striking, but ultimately not surprising, that this same phenomenon occurs via telemedicine as well.

One of the interesting parallels between Urgent Care Telemedicine and the ER is that we have recently been using scribes on our calls. They listen in on my consults, I tell them of any pertinent findings, the diagnosis, medications, and any other needed follow-up, and they put that all into the chart, making the encounter quicker and more efficient.

Having scribes has always been one of my pleasures in the ER, and I am finding a similar pleasure in having them as I do in telemedicine. Most of the scribes are pre-med, soon to apply to med school, and when we have time, we can discuss the many medical issues of the patients we "see" and my perspective on the larger issues in the world of medicine that they will be encountering as they move ahead. I recently worked with a scribe, and we immediately became very busy, as well as having problems with the telemedicine platform. This got me going on a rant about the many issues I have with medicine, and I asked her if she had seen an article from the New York Times documenting at great length the array of issues confronting and thwarting MDs in their attempts to provide time and uncompromised quality care to their patients. She'd not seen it, and I hesitated to forward it to her because it might dissuade her from moving ahead with her plans.

She disagreed, and rightly so. Said that she needed to know the reality of the situation as she did move ahead. This occasioned me to talk about my feelings at this point in my life and career.

After thirty-two years, I had been delighted to leave the ER behind, to begin work in urgent care. There, my thirty years of experience and expertise were in such demand, and I felt I was on top of my game, hyper-focused, and able to separate the wheat from the chaff, as it were. Knowing which patients were potentially very sick and needed to go to the ER, which ones I could turn around: someone with an early kidney infection or bad strep throat I could plug an IV into, give antibiotics fluids, steroids, all that I had in my bag of tricks from the ER and help them avoid that trip to the hospital. Sometimes, if it wasn't busy, I could do the precise plastic surgical work on their lacerations that I loved and were among the most gratifying things I'd do. I developed a coterie of like-minded buddies. It was a great experience to be with other docs who were "cowboys" in the best sense of the word. Having seen so much in our combined years in the ER, we walked into any patient encounter confident in our competence (and not afraid to consult a colleague when not sure).

As I now said to the scribe, forty-plus years into a multifaceted career in medicine, I was finding that my frustrations with the bureaucracy, the rapacious, unethical pharmaceutical cartels, the criminal insurance companies whose last concern is patient care, and the increasingly monopolistic hospital groups that can't seem to efficiently create timely patient access to practitioners (all of which have led to the explosion of the urgent cares that have employed me for the last ten years). It has all plunged me into a place of tension and unease.

Yet, I told her I still love what I do. I have helped steer potentially ill patients to get the urgent, and sometimes emergent, care they didn't realize they needed when they made an online appointment. And more generally, telemedicine is a pleasant gig. Many of the patient issues are straightforward and easily fixed. Neither the patient nor I needed to have schlepped anywhere for this encounter to have been carried out. Instead, we have our interaction from the quiet of our homes (or, on more than one occasion, their cars). I very much enjoy my ability to help people and take as much time as possible to explain things online. I realize that at this point in my life, doing online medical encounters is a comfortable way to continue my career. In short, I'm extremely fortunate that I have been able to have the opportunity to do it, to have consciously and not, reached this point in my profession and life.

To be able, at age seventy-six, to continue to learn and help and make people feel better is a truly humbling and gratifying thing, and I need to keep that in mind when obstacles try to get in the way.

CHAPTER 39

THE TRUTH ABOUT WEED

In the Fall of 2015, I was attending the monthly forum of Physicians for a National Health Program, sitting with a friend and former partner at Holy Name. As the forum was ending, and almost as an afterthought, Oscar turned to me and said, "Kenny, you know New York State is about to legalize medical cannabis!"

I didn't know, had missed that memo.

"Are you interested in registering with the state and starting a business to treat patients with weed?"

After a moment of reflection, I told him I certainly was. I initially found this proposed endeavor amusing because a few years before this, I'd been seeing a woman in L.A. who'd suggested on numerous occasions that I should reinstate my California medical license and spend time out there being a pot doc. I wasn't ready to make the move, our relationship was fraught, and part of the idea seemed flaky. I didn't like the idea of sitting in some *ferkakte* office as a line of "patients," many just looking to get stoned, rolled in. And I didn't want, in a rote, assembly line manner, to give them each a "scrip" to purchase cannabis. It also didn't help that, around that same time, there'd been a Man on the Street interview on the Jimmy Kimmel Show that I'd caught. It occurred in downtown LA and was conducted with people who'd just gotten their medical marijuana cards. Everyone had a different reason for why they needed it, some more plausible than others. But the one person that stuck out, when asked why she was getting a card, replied, "Oh, children, job...life!"

It was a funny and ultimately truthful response (as I have come to discover, now that I am ten years into certifying patients in New York) but at the time it seemed like more of a joke.

At that point, a few years after the Kimmel episode, with Oscar and my mutually acknowledged interest, and the excitement we felt about being part of a new, unfolding medical adventure, we decided to move ahead. Oscar also suggested that another friend, Neal (who I knew from the world of urgent care) join us in setting up the practice.

Neal signed on and the three of us immediately took the requisite 4-hour course to become registered certifiers with New York State. We formed a group I named Cannabis Doctors of New York (a name that turned out to be a fabulous marketing tool) and started seeing patients.

As we began, knowing that many of our patients might be disabled/homebound, we advertised that we would do house calls. Not long thereafter we were contacted by the husband of a woman who was looking for a home visit. I was available and soon found myself in the apartment of a lovely couple on the Upper East Side of Manhattan. After I sat and spoke with them and explained all I could about the benefits of medical cannabis and how the licensing process worked, the husband approached me and suggested that we should consider an entrepreneurial arrangement. Herb (a funny name in the cannabis world) could use his business and advertising skills, as well as his many connections, to help us jumpstart the practice.

After talking with Oscar and Neal, we decided to give it a try. Susan, my life partner who I consult with on most everything, was not overly enthusiastic (and in retrospect foresaw many of the issues that later developed), but I went along with my new partners and Herb came on board.

We started working out of his office and because of his connections, he soon found a woman to work with us as our representative and as the general face of the business. Marika had grown up with a father who'd been a grower/dealer of pot for years in California, she was now at Baruch studying business and was delighted to join us. She had great energy, was very smart, tuned in to the politics of cannabis, and was a tremendous asset. With her help we began navigating the evolving world of medically approved cannabis and all its attendant players and events, both educational and celebratory.

Early on, Susan, who when she is driving is either listening to Howard Stern or Doctor Radio (oh, and sometimes MSNBC), heard Dr. Julie Holland interviewed on the Dr. Billy show on Doctor Radio. Julie is a psychiatrist and among the vast array of things she has accomplished, she had recently edited *The Pot Book*. She was also interviewed by Dr. Sanjay Gupta for the three-part series he did on the benefits of cannabis. I was able to contact Julie, and she soon became a friend and advisor. Plus, it turned out she had an office space that she shared which was available to us. It was a perfect opportunity, and we began seeing patients there (as well as continuing to take advantage of Herb's office availability).

Marika, Susan, and I became immersed in the crescendo-like energy and the many functions occurring at this time in the burgeoning New York cannabis space. And, around this time, I hired Dani Sondrol, who'd done all the IT/computer work for my brother Neil's acupuncture practice, to put up our website and continually revamp it, use her great skills for PowerPoint presentations, and keep a watchful eye out for any of the multitude of ongoing online shenanigans a site and practice like ours could fall prey to.

Within the first year after the law went into effect, this space began exploding. People from across the socioeconomic spectrum, long-time surreptitious stoners, buttoned-up attorneys, and a select group of MDs seemed to emerge from the shadows. We loved being part of it, going out in the pre-COVID-19 world of NYC gatherings, meeting all the other people who were willing to take the plunge, getting to know like-minded individuals, and advocating for medical cannabis. What was interesting as well was that it soon became clear that not only were most of my medical colleagues uninterested in becoming involved with cannabis, but their ignorance of the medical benefits of the plant was, and is, striking. As much as anything else I attribute this to the fact that only 11% of United States medical schools teach about the Endocannabinoid System, or ECS. This system refers to the vast array of chemical transmitters, receptors, and pathways they stimulate, located throughout the brain and the rest of the body that mediate the effects that occur when using the plant. I suspect that my colleagues, like many others, are still influenced by the perennially successful 1930s propaganda film, Reefer Madness.

Meanwhile, Herb, who was a member of the Friars Club, suggested we use that venue to put on an event. We set up a lunch to be followed by an informational presentation on medical cannabis. The presenters that day were my partners Neal and Oscar, Julie, Richard Gottfried, the State Assemblyman who for eighteen years had been trying to get medical cannabis legislation passed (along with legislation to provide single-payer healthcare in New York. He and I met in the past through PNHP on that issue); Nick Vita, the CEO of the Columbia Care dispensary and his head pharmacist, Tricia Reed. It was incredibly well attended, got some nice publicity for us, for medical cannabis and The Friars, and helped establish our groups' medical cannabis bona fides in New York.

I was next asked to speak on a panel for Women Grow (a national organization dedicated to ensuring that women had full access to and opportunities in, the cannabis space). After the panel, I was approached by Dr. Richard Carlton, a brilliant psychiatrist well versed in the biochemistry of cannabis and someone who I discovered subsequently was long accustomed to advocacy and working outside of the box. A few years prior, when the Compassionate Care Act (the law legalizing medical cannabis in New York) was being debated, Richard had been involved in advocating for its legalization, speaking in front of the state legislature. He was interested in joining our group, and we were happy, as non-psychiatrists, to get him on board. We were well aware of the tricky and treacherous emotional responses that develop in some patients exposed to cannabis, and we were glad to have someone to refer to for any of our patients who had potential or pre-existing psychiatric issues.

Not long after that we gave a dinner along with a very well attended presentation at The Players Club in Gramercy Park. On the panel, in addition to Oscar, Tricia, and myself, we had Marvin Washington, a former New York Jet. Marvin is a strong advocate for medical cannabis, and he spoke about how many of his teammates would use cannabis before games because they realized it was much better for pain and inflammation than narcotics. I have to say, I never asked Marvin how being stoned affected their abilities on the field, but I do know that, depending on the strain, cannabis can tremendously help one's focus, energy, and physicality. (I've been told that Arnold Schwarzenegger always got stoned before a workout). Plus, Marvin and his teammates were aware of the research showing cannabis could help prevent TBI (traumatic brain injury), a condition they knew many of them could fall prey to.

We also became part of the annual Cannabis World Expo run by Christine Ianuzzi, at Javits Center. We began speaking on the educational panels and getting a booth on the large convention floor to showcase Cannabis Doctors of New York. The third year we were there, Herb, Neal, and Oscar departed Cannabis Doctors, and everything was in great flux. We had already purchased a booth though, and Susan suggested we give it to a couple we'd just met. They both worked in the theatre and were trying to get the show Reefer Madness produced. It was a perfect way for them to get their names out there and we were happy to give the booth to them.

It was a terrible blow to lose my partners, and I found myself (without much business acumen) suddenly totally in charge of what had become a well-established business and brand. With Susan's help, I gradually reorganized the practice.

And I brought a new person, Lauren Beshara, on board to help with patient care issues. She has become the warm, compassionate voice (and so much more) of Cannabis Doctors of New York, keeping the practice running smoothly. Through a widening referral base of patients, MDs (who are happy to refer us difficult patients for whom nothing else has worked), and Adult Living Communities, I've been fairly busy. In fact, I now have a cannabis nurse as part of the practice. Sarah Halweil, extremely experienced, knowledgeable, and compassionate, has become a valued member of the team, adding her unique perspective as we navigate the world of caring for the wide array of patients we are seeing.

As occurred in other states, Adult Use, now legal in New York, has occasioned a sharp decline in medical patients as many people believe they can self-medicate without input from practitioners, or the pharmacists New York

State mandates must be seen before getting access to medical cannabis.

And yet, a decade in, I'm seeing patients, advocating for medical cannabis, and lecturing at various venues, including each year to the family practice residents at Northwell and to CaringKind (a major advocacy group in New York for patients with Alzheimer's Disease and their caregivers).

As I try to assess things at this point, I think of the many patients I've certified and continue to see after five, six, seven, or eight years and how often they will say, "Cannabis has been a game changer for me."

"I wish someone would have told me about this years ago."

"I've been taking it for my chronic pain but realized it was really helpful in dealing with my anxiety as well!"

I think of my patient, MR, who has a long history of seizures, documented grand and petit mal, who, over three years, has either decreased or discontinued the dose of the prior seizure medications he was on, while simultaneously decreasing the number of seizures he has up to twenty a month down to three or four (all in consultation with his neurologist).

Or my patient, EF, a very successful finance person with chronic pain, who has found the "sweet spot" in his dosing of cannabis during the day. When I asked if being in that groove, as he described it, his pain abated from cannabis, allowed him to focus on the ongoing complicated financial transactions he has to perform, he said,

"Absolutely. It removes my concerns about pain and lets me focus on exactly what I am doing at work."

We discussed how having found the sweet spot allowed him greater calm and removed the emotional component of the pain. He knows he has something reliable to use when the pain is an issue that doesn't have the potential side effects other traditional meds have and that allows him to have greater productivity.

Another thing I have realized is that having access to medical cannabis, in its many forms and varying ratios of THC/CBD and other components of the plant, allows patients to have autonomy in how they treat their various medical conditions. After an initial lengthy consultation with me and a meeting with a pharmacist, patients can begin to see what works (or doesn't) for them. The patients I have who do the best (and from follow-up interviews, I'd estimate this happens for at least 70% of them) are the ones who take their time, jot down notes on their response to different formulations, and gradually weave cannabis into their daily lives. This thoughtful use of cannabis brings them back to the way things had been before they developed the medical condition that brought them to me. In a time when the paternalistic world of medicine is under scrutiny (rightfully I believe), it is refreshing and gratifying as a practitioner to have this very different ongoing relationship with the patients I now have.

One added benefit is that I've gotten referrals for patients from my brother Neil. He still lives in Ithaca, and was, until recently, an Acupuncture and Oriental Medicine practitioner there. It has been a great new way to bond with Neil and share our ideas and understanding of disease (which we never did as much of when I was practicing more traditional Western medicine).

As I've developed a more nuanced understanding of how the plant and our ECS interact I realize that in many ways, 40 years later, I've come full circle to the issues I was most interested in when I started my career in medicine. I've begun to see how cannabis works in very subtle, but also profound ways, how the vast pathways of the ECS (the master system of neurotransmitters) and its diffuse connections to the other neurotransmitter systems, allow it to help in so many disease states affecting all organ systems. This plant and its hundreds of different compounds is the only one I know of that can lower seizure frequency, decrease the inflammation of autoimmune diseases, lessen acute and chronic pain, and help the muscle spasticity of Multiple Sclerosis, to name a few of its attributes.

And so now I see this as the perfect return to what had always interested me in medicine and perceive the ECS as a great roadmap or lens, a spelunker's guide to the caverns and connections in the brain/mind.

One day, after being once again provoked to understand the array of benefits I was seeing with so many of my patients, I had an epiphany: I decided that the ECS mediated the placebo effect. I immediately decided that I was brilliant and that this was a groundbreaking realization until I went online and discovered that not only had other practitioners had this thought, but some had published scholarly papers on it. One in particular looked in-depth at connections between the ECS and the brain's various endorphin receptors and gave a plausible and extremely well-thought-out explanation for why placebo effects could be mediated by the ECS.

Recently, the OCM (Office of Cannabis Management, the state agency mandated to run the medical cannabis program) sponsored the First Symposium on Medical Cannabis with Roswell Park Institute in Buffalo. It was very well-attended and brought together practitioners and academics throughout the state. The next Symposium will be in November of 2025, in conjunction with the Northwell Cannabis Research group I'm a part of. I see this as a critical piece of what needs to be done to move things forward: working with legitimate, well-respected medical institutions to educate our colleagues, the media, legislators, and the public, about the benefits, and risks, of medical cannabis.

After ten years, there is a core group of us who persevere. I've now seen about 1,500 patients and gotten deeply involved with a community both national and international. I am constantly provoked emotionally and intellectually by my patient encounters and what I learn as I go deeper and deeper into this space,

Recently, I've been most excited and touched by my work with elderly patients with dementia and associated behavioral issues. With another colleague in New York and one in California, we've been seeing remarkable benefits from various strains of cannabis to help with anxiety-induced aggression and have even seen some cognitive improvements. Working with others I've been able to help children with autism as well, a tremendously gratifying thing to be able to accomplish at this point in my career.

I feel enormously fortunate to be stimulated constantly, to collaborate with others who are as excited as I am, working with and learning about this plant. It's a plant that I believe we, as homo sapiens have evolved with over countless millennia and which I believe holds tremendous promise in the coming years.

Recently, I was asked to see an elderly woman with crippling anxiety who was drinking two bottles of wine a day. Working with my colleague Sang Choi, then head pharmacist at the Etain dispensary, we began her on a regimen that quickly melted her anxiety away, and her alcohol consumption decreased to, at most, a glass of wine with dinner. Now, over two years later, she and her family are extremely pleased with how her life has turned around.

I must finally mention a patient I was seeing, a Hasidic Jew with Inflammatory Bowel Disease. He'd gotten permission from his rebbe to use cannabis for a disease that standard medicine wasn't helping much. He soon found a product that was quite helpful for his IBD. One day not long thereafter I was doing a follow-up with him, and he said, "Doctor. I have a question. Can THC give you wisdom?"

This intrigued me and I asked what he meant.

"Well," he said. "I've been studying Talmud all my life, but I find that when I take my THC and then look at passages in it, I know so well, I see them in a different, and deeper, way. And it's not because I'm stoned. I've talked to the rebbe and my wife about this and they agree my insights are valid!"

All of these stories and observations and the obvious benefits are so gratifying to me at this point in my life. I feel good knowing that I am involved with something that I can continue pursuing as long as I have the energy and focus to explore the vast possibilities this plant has to offer us.

Recently, I spoke to a man who is not just a rabbi and a moyl, but a physician as well.

In the course of our long conversation, he stated, "This plant has been with us forever. And from my deep research into it, I believe that the Burning Bush was cannabis."

I had to laugh at this observation but realized I couldn't argue with him about it either.

CHAPTER 40

The Little Nowhere of the Mind

My grandfather, Mischa Weinberg, made house calls. He had emigrated from Russia in the early 1900s, put himself through Fordham Medical School by working as a motorman on the BMT subway, done his internship at Beth Israel Hospital in Newark, and then, in the summer of 1920, set up a practice as a general practitioner in that New Jersey city. He would see patients at the office in the front of his home during the morning, do his hospital rounds and then, every afternoon, he would get into his battered Packard sedan to visit sick and injured families in their homes in the predominately Jewish and later Black communities of that resilient, ever-changing metropolis. It was a routine he continued until 1963, the year he died.

My great uncle, Marvin (supposedly the first baby ever delivered by Mischa), whose family spent a lot of time at Mischa's home in Newark, had told me years ago that after going out on his calls my grandfather would come home late in the evening to his wife and four children, and frequently a cold supper as well, put his hand in his pocket and pull out wads of crumpled one and five dollar bills, money taken from those who could afford to pay (family lore had it that he never charged those who couldn't).

Forty-five years later, after being an emergency medicine physician for twenty-five years, I found myself following in Mischa's footsteps, seeing homebound elderly patients in Bergen County, New Jersey, and treating foreign tourists in New York City who required acute medical care. Having begun this second medical career at the age of 59, no longer married, daughter away at college, I would come home late from my calls to an empty apartment, no food in the fridge, and the only bills coming from my pocket were insurance forms to be sent in for reimbursement.

One of these house calls took place on a sunny fall afternoon when I was notified about a patient who needed to be seen for pain in his left heel. I drove to the Upper West Side of Manhattan, entered a large building on West End Avenue, and was met at the apartment door by a retired Scottish gastroenterologist. He and his wife, also a retired MD, had just flown to New York City to see their newborn grandchild and were staying in the spacious, bright, pre-war apartment of their son and daughter-in-law. The previous day, my patient and his wife had taken a bus tour to Greenwich Village, then decided to walk back uptown. On the morning I saw him, he had awakened with severe pain in the back of his foot. Unsure of what was causing his problem, he had called his insurance company to get medical help. He recounted this all to me when I arrived, and after examining him, I found I didn't have a clear answer to his problem either. I was concerned, however, that after his long walk, he could have a fracture, so I made arrangements for an X-ray to be taken later in the day. When I left, I told him I'd let him know as soon as I received the results, and we would make a treatment plan from there.

That evening, I got the radiologists' reading. My patient's pain was caused not by a fracture but by a bony outgrowth of the heel bone—a calcaneal "spur." I called him and discussed the treatment—steroids injected into the area of the calcaneus, which I could do the following day.

When I arrived that afternoon, I began my ministrations by drawing up my medication into a syringe. He lay prone on the bed, his wife placed towels under his leg in the makeshift surgical suite we arranged in the guest bedroom, and then he bent his knee and lifted his foot. As I scrubbed the heel with antiseptic, numbed it, and then injected the steroids we plunged back into a conversation from the day before about a shared interest in literature, and writing we had done, and he mentioned that a piece of his had just been published in *British Medical Journal* (BMJ). The article was a review of a book, *Tea with Walter de la Mare*, written by the British neurologist Lord Brain (a man whose name seemed to leave little doubt as to what his calling in life would be), talking of the relationship that developed between two men of differing backgrounds: Brain, the renowned British physician and de la Mare, a poet and writer of fiction and essays on mind and spirit. I had heard of Lord Russell Brain, barely, but I drew a blank on de la Mare.

I wrapped up the foot, and our literary discussion told my patient to call if there were any problems, and went home, nearly forgetting about the encounter. But something about what he had said piqued my curiosity and not long afterward I found and read his article in the BMJ, tracked him down online and we began to correspond via email. I investigated and discovered that Brain, knighted for his many accomplishments in medicine (his textbook, *Brain Diseases of the Nervous System* was standard reading for medical students in the UK for many years) was also very interested in the mind and psyche. He had come upon a book of de la Mare's that contained an essay on the Bloomsbury poet Rupert Brooke in which Brooke had used the phrase "the little nowhere of the mind," referring to that ineluctable region between mind and body.

When Brain saw that phrase, he "recognized a fellow spirit," as my Scottish patient put it, and tried to locate the quote but couldn't find it in any of Brooke's poetry. He contacted de la Mare and during that writer's investigation (during which it turned out the phrase was actually "the little nowhere of the brain"), a correspondence developed. Not long afterward, in the early 1950s, Brain and de la Mare moved into the town of Twickenham in southwest London. De la Mare invited Brain for Sunday tea and over several years the two met and a friendship developed as they discussed topics such as painting, literature, ghosts, and not surprisingly, the realms between mind and body.

My patient had come upon Brain's account of this relationship in the book "Tea with de la Mare" (including the fact that Brain had been invited to see de la Mare for a last chat the night before the poet died) and was so taken by, as he said, "the privilege to eavesdrop on the private conversations of such men" that he had written his article about it in the British journal.

All of this ruminated in my brain for a month or so and then I realized I had to pursue these titillating tidbits. I read Wikipedia and other online references to Brain, de la Mare, and Brooke; found myself ordering Tea with Walter de la Mare, long out of print (though an original edition was available); learned that not only had Brain been a pre-eminent neurologist, an editor of the journal Brain, and had a reflex named after him, but that he had written extensively about medical aspects of the work of authors such as Dickens, Swift, and Samuel Johnson.

Intrigued, I researched further and learned all I could about de la Mare. I found that not only was he a poet but also a writer of books for children as well as adults, including one published in 1922, Memoirs of a Midget. I subsequently bought that book (not an original edition) and while immersed in reading about the life of a very small young woman began wondering if, since Memoirs predated by a few years, Stuart Little, E.B. White could have been influenced by it (in subsequent correspondence with someone who knew White, I was told that even though White had most likely read Memoirs, his book was purely autobiographical).

Because of de la Mare's interest in matters of philosophy and spirituality he had written an essay in his book, Pleasures and Speculation, which contained the phrase by Rupert Brooke that was the pebble in the pond whose ripple first reached Brain, then my patient, and ultimately, nearly 100 years later, me.

But if I had thought Brain or de la Mare were interesting and current when I looked into Rupert Brooke I was astonished by the fact this man, described by William Butler Yeats as "the handsomest young man in England" at the turn of the last century; an athlete and academic who won a scholarship to Cambridge; quoted extensively by the British for his "war" poetry (though his warrior ethos seemed questionable at best); and buried in a lonely and haunting, dutifully marked grave on a hillside on the Greek island of Spyros (he died aboard a naval ship in the Mediterranean during WWI) had created many more ripples than just the one that resonated with me. His line "Well this side of Paradise...there's little comfort in the wise" inspired F. Scott Fitzgerald; his poetry was quoted by Radar on the TV series, "MASH"; included in lyrics by Pink Floyd and Fleetwood Mac; and as recently as 1981, sixty-six years after his death, the movie, Making Love with Kate Jackson used his work, naming the child born to Jackson's character after him.

While most of my house calls are of a more mundane and less engaging nature than this one, never before, or since, sending me on such a literary and intellectual odyssey, or allowing me to see fine scholarly distinctions among my friends (only one even knew who Rupert Brooke was and—something I'd just discovered myself—that he had gone skinny dipping with Virginia Woolf) I did began to wonder if Mischa ever had had this kind of experience with his house call patients.

One of the remaining relatives who knew my grandfather well was my father's youngest brother Martin. While speaking of his father recently, Martin told me that as a youngster he would sit in the car waiting when his father did many of his house calls and how, one hot summer night after watching his father trudge down from a third-floor walk-up he asked if he had been paid for the visit. He was told by Mischa, "If they say 'Doc, how much do I owe you,' I'll tell them a price I know they can afford. If they don't ask as I'm heading towards the door, I know they have no money, and I won't bring the subject up."

Though I was brought up knowing my grandfather was a Talmudic scholar turned atheist I don't get a sense of whether he ever had the time or interest to pursue these types of literary expeditions. My feeling is he had barely a moment to do more than schlep up and down the stairs in the apartments of the working-class families he was serving; provide them with the excellent care I heard about from others when I was growing up; take their crumpled dollars, or not; and treat them with the compassion and wisdom I remember him showing me when he fought my recurrent childhood bouts of tonsillitis, giving me penicillin injections on many occasions, and refusing, correctly, to allow my tonsils to be taken out. So, while he probably never was spurred by a patient visit to explore the type of ground I've been covering I'm certain he walked out of most of his encounters feeling satisfied, feeling he had helped someone; by dint of his personality and compassion and expertise had made someone feel better or have less pain.

That is what we share. It is what bridges the gap between our generations and years and the grave and gives my trips to patients' homes an added, deeply enriching poignancy.

POSTSCRIPT

I recently reunited with my cousin, Tommy Weinberg, my Uncle Arthur's son and the oldest of Mischa's grandchildren. He had spent a lot of time with Mischa growing up (especially on the farm Mischa had in then rural Freehold, New Jersey) and has been able to color in a much clearer picture of my grandfather. From him, I learned that Mischa was (not surprisingly) an avid reader who plied Tom with an array of books and medical articles through his adolescence. What struck me most and again should not have surprised me in the least, was that Mischa was most drawn to books written by physicians, especially those who wrote about their own experiences as patients.

Tommy also remembered that Mischa had died in bed with a book beside him.

It seems that perhaps that thread from the Baal Shem Tov to Mischa, Clepe, and then to me was even stronger than I know.

ACKNOWLEDGMENTS

This book has been a long time in the making. During my forty-plus-year career in medicine, I have been interviewed on television and radio and had many pieces of my writing published, but most of my time has revolved around working in the ER, and later, making house calls and practicing urgent care medicine. It all felt routine, a predictable path, not something to spend time chronicling. I would never have considered writing a memoir. My life hadn't felt particularly worthy of being elevated to that status.

While I had started writing a bit during my first career in film, the need to document and make sense of what I was now immersed in began in earnest when I wound up working in the ER at Bellevue and New York University Hospital. I would come home from my shifts there (and then throughout the rest of my medical career) clutching "snippets", notes of various lengths, capturing the array of characters and moments I'd just experienced. When I had time and inclination, I'd flesh them out into actual stories.

After I had written a few stories and wanted feedback, I shared them with those closest to me, including my dear friend, Bella Meyer. Notably, her critique occurred on a tumultuous day in 2001 in Washington, D.C. Her husband Martin Kace, a successful business executive, branding *macher*, and human rights advocate, critically injured and now wheelchair-bound, had organized a protest in front of the U.S. Capitol. Congress was voting that day on whether to fund stem cell research. It was felt that stem cells held tremendous promise in treating spinal cord injuries and then, as now, religious conservatives were fighting to prevent the funding. Martin felt that he needed to stage a forceful and compelling protest. He had assembled four other wheelchair-bound paraplegics, and all five of them were positioned under separate free-standing gallows on the Capitol lawn. Press and bystanders assembled nearby. Martin had set things up so that on his command the five paralyzed men would be yanked out of their wheelchairs and hung from the gallows, symbolizing what would happen to them if the funding wasn't passed and their situations were not addressed. I was asked to be there, in my white ER doctor coat, both for visual impact and should anything untoward occur during the event. The vote failed, and not many years thereafter, sadly, Martin died from complications of his injury.

Later that same day, however, Bella offered her thoughtful critiques of my stories, and she and Martin subsequently, as a birthday gift, enrolled me in a creative writing course at NYU. The course was run by poet and writer, Peggy Garrison, who was delighted to have an MD in the mix of students. Thanks to Peggy, I learned about a first-time retreat for medical writers and poets, "Writing the Medical Experience." It was to be hosted by the prestigious Community of Writers (then called "Squaw Valley Community of Writers"). I submitted two pieces, was accepted, and that summer, found myself in the company of Drs. Richard Selzer, Danielle Ofri, and Frank Huyler, among others. That experience and being part of that community was transformational and solidified my commitment to, and great pleasure in, writing.

More recently, having written over twenty-five stories, several of which had made it into print, I decided to assemble them into a book and reached out to various literary agents and publishers without success. I ultimately decided to self-publish and needed an editor to help guide me through the process.

I was eventually introduced to Gay Walley, who is not only an editor but also, a novelist and screenwriter. Gay read my pieces and sensed that they were part of a larger project: all that I alluded to, my backstory, was really the basis for a medical memoir.

With her help, I wrote this book, weaving together important events in my life with the short stories I'd written when those events were occurring. She also suggested I send the chapter I subsequently wrote, musing on the deep connections between literature and medicine, to *Psychology Today*. Not long thereafter, I was contacted by the editor there, who was intrigued by the piece and invited me to do a blog. A year and a half later, my blog, "Bedside Manners," (thank you, Susan, for that title) has had nine posts, close to 50,000 views, and the post I did recently on "Cannabis and the Elderly" immediately resulted in my being contacted by the head of the New York State Department of Aging, who arranged a livestream with him on the topic.

When Gay suggested doing the memoir, I was initially hesitant. Yet, as I wrote the additional chapters, aided tremendously by the journals, diaries, and dream books (as I've variously called them) that I've been keeping since college, I developed a different perspective on my seventy-six years.

Interestingly, all but one of those journals survive. The one that doesn't was stolen from the back of our VW beetle, *Tortuguita* (Little Turtle), along with so many other valuables late one night in Guadalajara. My brother, Marc, and I awoke in the morning to find the car trashed but drivable, as we took off, as first-year med students, for a week of treating *campesinos* (poor Mexican families) residing in rural villages outside of Guadalajara. The stolen journal contained my evolving thoughts as I made the transition from working in film to deciding to be a physician, documenting a pivotal time in my life that led to all that has occurred since.

Speaking of Marc, I want to thank both my brothers, Neil and Marc. Marc was one of the funniest, smartest, and most loving people I have ever known. He died much too young. Our time together in "God, What A Horror" (Guadalajara, thank you, "Nails" Nathan) bound us together in the most profound, disturbing, and riotous ways. His understanding of medicine and healing was monumental, and I know it greatly influenced both Neil and me. (When he died, his wife, Ruth, stepped in and took his place as the Third Musketeer to me and Neil.) Neil, who fortunately is quite alive and well, is a gentle, kind, and creative man. He is the one I go to for his expertise in all things related to horticulture, ornithology, and the washtub bass. I think, as the middle brother, he felt comfortable and protected enough to delve into and share his explorations in music, yoga, photography, acupuncture, and herbal medicine long before I had a clue.

Throughout my life, I have maintained close relationships with colleagues, friends, and family. Cousin James Treuhaft was my first buddy and playmate. Smart, talented, and always needing to push limits, we've shared many adventures, several of which I'm glad we made it out of alive. In kindergarten, I met Kenneth R. Weissberg or "Schickie". (I call him that because early on in our friendship, my father started referring to him as *Schiklegrubr*, Adolf Hitler's original name.) I needn't get into that reference more here, but we have a seventy-year history of hilarious and not-so experiences, Eastern European accents, and memories, any of which can be called up in an instant and that form a repertoire we've long referred to as "Inspired Insanity".

Speaking of inspiration, I want to thank my mentor and friend of over forty years, Dr. Lewis Goldfrank. Not only did I learn a tremendous amount from him during my time at NYU, but he also recognized early on my interest in ethics and writing and provided me the opportunity to hone my skills in those areas. I've been sending Lewis my stories over the years, and he graciously offered to write the foreword to this book.

I also want to thank Dr. Oli Fein, who counseled me amid a crisis I was having many years into my career as an emergency physician. Because of my writing, he introduced me to Dr. Rita Charon, who'd taken his position at Columbia when Oli left to become a dean at Weill Cornell. Rita had recently established the Program in Narrative Medicine at the College of Physicians and Surgeons, and we immediately developed a bond. I plunged into several roles there, which gave a new meaning and depth to my life and writing.

My daughter, Georgia, my *veldt* (world) over the last thirty-four years, is a constant source of joy and *nachas*. As a very young girl, she would ask me to tell her ER stories before she went to sleep. So many years later, she now amazes and amuses me with her creativity, grit, and highly conceptualized and enchanting understanding of life. My ex-wife and Georgia's biological mother was an early supporter of my writing and is a thoughtful, loving co-parent.

I want to express my deepest gratitude to Susan, my pragmatic muse and inspiration, who is extremely encouraging and supportive of my writing. She is thoughtful, protective, creative, and the *yin* to my *yang*. Despite her joking about her tendency to "pick fly shit out of pepper," she has contributed countless invaluable edits and numerous title suggestions.

Most importantly, her genuine concern for my well-being when I'm not paying attention has literally saved my life, as well as helped me avoid potentially treacherous business decisions. I might have succumbed not long ago to a totally asymptomatic aortic aneurysm that was discovered by the new PCP she wisely suggested I see when I turned seventy.

Lastly, my parents: My mother had a wicked, ironic sense of humor, a love of literature, words, and grammar (I can't remember how many times she corrected me when I used who instead of whom). She was deeply engaged in a lifelong exploration of painting, drawing, collage, and construction, and most critically, her love of me, Neil, and Marc supplied a bedrock of support and encouragement to explore and create for my brothers and me.

As I was writing this book, I had the realization that my father, also such a force, such a significant presence in my life, had three times used a remarkably similar phrase at critical points in his life and mine: "Kenny, I want you to show you something," when, the day before my scheduled examination at the Newark (New Jersey) draft board, he handed me a psychiatrist's letter that he had clearly dictated to the shrink. I read the three-page handwritten narrative in amazement. The next day, May 20, 1970, on my twenty-second birthday, I gave this missive to the Army psychiatrist. As he read it, it became clear that I would never be selected to serve in the deadly and deceit-plagued Vietnam War. (It was so damning that I didn't get the 4-F I'd expected but was classified 1-Y, only eligible to be called up in the event of a nuclear war.)

"Kenny, listen to my heart," when, at age thirty-two, at home with my mother and brothers to celebrate the start of my medical internship, he handed me a gift. With great pleasure, I pulled out the new Littman Cardiology stethoscope and put it to his chest. To my great dismay, I immediately heard the murmur he already knew he had, letting us know, in his way, that he was going to need open heart surgery in the near future. (This, of course, resonated with me thirty-eight years later when my physician told me about the heart murmur he'd just heard, alerting me about that asymptomatic aortic aneurysm I was walking around with and that needed to be repaired.) Finally, "Kenny, I want you to feel something," requested of me three days before he died. He asked me to touch a wound on his arm as the blood oozed out cold, a manifestation of the bone marrow failure that soon would kill him.

Writing this, weaving together my stories and my story has been therapeutic to me as I near my seventy-seventh birthday. I've been fortunate to reach this age in good health (*kina hora*), having accomplished what I have, carrying on the Weinberg family tradition of healing and caring, and being surrounded by the love of family and friends. And here, I would like to mention Ruth and my late brother, Marc's daughter, Sara, now the fourth generation of Weinbergs to carry on that MD tradition.

I hope that all comes through in this book: caring, healing, humility, love, and humor. A good prescription for a satisfying life.

Finally, I am grateful to Candi S. Cross. When I was hitting roadblocks, trying to get this published through "conventional channels" and being told that a medical memoir wasn't commercially interesting, I met her. She has helped tie up all the loose editorial ends, delivered a book cover and finished product I'm very happy with, and shepherded it across the finish line with a lot of early praise.

ABOUT THE AUTHOR

Kenneth Weinberg, born into a family of physicians and humanitarian relatives passionate about politics, literature, humor, and art, developed a unique blend of interests. His education and career took shape during the tumultuous '60s and '70s, first as he pursued undergraduate studies at the University of Wisconsin, Madison, earning a degree in Television and Film Production and then, working in that field for four years. However, having grown up with a father and grandfather as doctors and a mother as an artist, he was compelled to channel his creativity into his longstanding interest in mind/body medicine and decided to become a physician.

Amid the social upheaval on college campuses, his passionate activism negatively affected his grades as an undergraduate; nevertheless, determined to follow this course, he and his youngest brother chose to pursue their medical education in Mexico, viewing this opportunity as a path for their future.

Having been accepted back in the United States to do a residency in Internal Medicine, at LA County-USC Medical Center, Weinberg returned to New York City for a Fellowship in Psychoneuroimmunology at the Manhattan VA. Regrettably, a study he had begun, which involved treating AIDS patients with acupuncture (in 1984), was quashed. This setback led him to embark on a remarkable 32-year career in emergency medicine, beginning at Bellevue Hospital.

During his tenure at Bellevue, Weinberg's writing career took off as he delved into ethical dilemmas, Munchausen's Syndrome, and the harrowing yet rewarding encounters he played a pivotal role in while treating patients in the ER. His activism and humanitarian background fueled his advocacy for serious healthcare reform while his creative impulses led him to participate in The Program in Narrative Medicine at Columbia University's College of Physicians and Surgeons.

Weinberg's career trajectory encompassed various settings, including house calls, urgent care, and, over the past ten years, as a medical cannabis practitioner. These diverse experiences have shaped his evolving career and contributed to his unique perspective on healthcare and literature. The humility and *Borscht Belt* sense of humor Weinberg brings to his writing is both infectious and curative.

www.ingramcontent.com/pod-product-compliance
Lightning Source LLC
LaVergne TN
LVHW102010210926
848483LV00015B/449/J